INJURIES IN SPORT

INJURIES IN SPORT

A guide for the accident department and general practice

DAVID SUTHERLAND MUCKLE
MB BS, MS, MD, FRCS

Consultant, Cleveland Area Health Authority, Middlesbrough General Hospital; North Tees Hospital; Research Associate, University of Durham; Surgeon, Middlesbrough A.F.C.; Formerly Adviser, Oxford United F.C., Oxford University F.C.; Medical Adviser to the Football Association and the F.I.F.A. in 'The World Football Development Programme'; Medical Instructor, F.I.F.A.

Second edition

WRIGHT·PSG

BRISTOL   LONDON   BOSTON
1982

© D. S. Muckle, 'Redcroft', 72 The Grove, Marton, Middlesbrough, Cleveland, TS7 8AJ. 1982

All Rights Reserved. No part of this publication may be reproduced, stored in a retrieval system, or transmitted in any form or by any means, electronic, mechanical, photocopying, recording or otherwise, without the prior permission of the Copyright owner.

Published by:
John Wright & Sons Ltd, 42–44 Triangle West, Bristol BS8 1EX, England
John Wright PSG Inc., 545 Great Road, Littleton, Massachusetts 01460, U.S.A.

First edition 1978
Reprinted 1980 (*twice*)
Second edition 1982

British Library Cataloguing in Publication Data

Muckle, David Sutherland
Injuries in sport.
1. Sports—Accidents and injuries
I. Title
617'.1027   RD131

ISBN 0 7236 0620 X

Library of Congress Catalog Card Number 81—70075

PRINTED IN GREAT BRITAIN BY HENRY LING LTD, A SUBSIDIARY OF JOHN WRIGHT AND SONS LTD, AT THE DORSET PRESS, DORCHESTER

Preface

The immediate success of this book has resulted in the demand for a second edition. Therefore, I have taken the opportunity to revise part of the text, to re-draw certain illustrations and add new material. With the recent increased participation by the public in sport at both amateur and professional levels, the medical profession has finally become interested in sports medicine. However, it is a broad subject encompassing applied physiology in relation to fitness, psychology, physiotherapy, rehabilitation and nutrition as well as the injury problems themselves. This book is concerned with the latter aspect of sports medicine as seen from the surgical point of view and is addressed to all doctors who are interested in sport, and especially those in Casualty, Orthopaedic and Rehabilitation Departments, as well as in General Practice. The text tends to concentrate on injuries that are relatively sports specific but occasionally there is bound to be an overlap with basic orthopaedic teaching. However, this has been kept to a minimum whenever possible by the use of line drawings, as for example in outlining fracture patterns. It is hoped that this new edition will continue to serve the same basic need as before, giving both an introduction to sports injuries while collating fundamental knowledge.

I appreciate permission given by the editors and contributors of the *Journal of Bone and Joint Surgery*, British and American Editions, *Injury*, *Orthopedic Clinics in North America*, *Medisport*, the *Physician & Sports Medicine*, and the *British Journal of Sports Medicine* to reproduce certain illustrations used in this book. I would also like to thank the staff of Messrs John Wright & Sons Ltd of Bristol; Margaret Stevenson and Pam Smith who checked the proofs; the Photographic Department of Middlesbrough General Hospital (Ken Goult); the Radiology Department of Middlesbrough General Hospital; and Julie Flounders, my Secretary, for her help in preparing the manuscript.

D.S.M.

Contents

1	Introduction	1
2	Frequency and site of injury	4
3	Immediate care	10
4	Soft-tissue injuries—acute	17
5	Soft-tissue injuries—chronic	36
6	Injuries to the thigh and knee	47
7	Meniscal damage in the knee	55
8	Ligamentous injuries in the knee	68
9	Injuries to the tibia, ankle and foot	83
10	Shoulder and upper limb injuries	101
11	Injuries to the head and face	121
12	Injuries to the spine	132
13	Chest, abdomen and pelvic injuries	139
14	Injuries to the skin	146

References 151

Index 157

Chapter 1

Introduction

It should be stated from the outset that in compiling this text the author has deliberately concentrated on injuries which can be considered as being 'sports specific'. It would be logical to call any injury occurring during a sporting event a 'sports injury' but this would involve such ramifications of subject material that eventually this book would resemble yet another orthopaedic or accident publication.

Since participation in and love of sport are an integral part of human behaviour and accidents are bound to happen, sport and medicine have become naturally complementary both in terms of fitness and therapy. But as the days have long since passed when natural skill alone was sufficient to secure success in sport so has the period when sports medicine can be carried out on a hobby basis with little or no firm scientific foundation and investigation. The treatment of the injured sportsman often requires special judgement and experience plus a commensurate knowledge of the sport involved. The Greek and Roman physicians recognized that supreme physical fitness was artificial in the sense that it was not inherent in the individual but had to be cultivated by months of dedicated effort. The same is true today and the sheer volume of time put into training by professional athletes is often quite remarkable—runners may complete 200 miles per week, swimmers may spend 4 or 5 hours in the water daily and the acquisition of skills for an event such as the pentathlon may utilize even longer periods per day. Thus the exploitation of athletic prowess can easily be disrupted by minor medical problems.

Sport is essentially a period of contrived play and since it involves physical activity it will give rise to physiological stress, the extent of the alteration in homeostatic balance depending on the period of adaptation (training) which has preceded it. It is common practice to divide sports into those with repetitive actions (e.g. running, swimming, rowing) which have injuries mainly of an intrinsic nature, i.e. self-inflicted and arising from specific incidents not involving an outside agency, and those sports in which the pattern of play is constantly changing (e.g. football, tennis, rugby) when extrinsic injuries are produced, i.e. caused by contact with an external object (another player, apparatus or vehicle).

Whatever sport is considered, the basic requirements of speed, strength, endurance and skill are common factors; each may be hampered by a prolonged absence through injury.

The effective management of a sports injury is easily divided into three interrelated phases: prevention, diagnosis and treatment.

PREVENTION

Rules are designed to protect the participants and it is essential that they are rigorously enforced by the referee or umpire. Even sports with no official rules such as mountaineering have well-recognized codes to protect the individual. Such self-control is essential both during competition and training. Faults in clothes and equipment need rectifying immediately they occur; and it is important that sportswear and protective clothing should be designed in consultation with medical advice, e.g. many of the modern cut-away football boots with poor studding and soles predispose to ankle injuries and their design runs contrary to medical thought.

DIAGNOSIS

This must be prompt and accurate, and since the nature and distribution of an injury tend to follow a set pattern of play (e.g. a collapse of the rugby scrum may cause ligamentous damage in the knee) some appreciation of the body's momentum during the period of injury is helpful in reaching a quick diagnosis.

TREATMENT

This should be logically prescribed against a background of accurate diagnosis. Any doctor interested in sports injuries soon learns that the treatment of a soft-tissue injury is a curious admixture of rest, body exercises and training which requires skilful judgement to maintain the fine balance between the immobilization of the injured part and the activity of the player as a whole. The principal aims of therapy are to restore full muscle power, extensibility, range of movements and skill patterns.

However, sports medicine is not just an amalgam of trauma, orthopaedics and general surgery carried out by an enthusiastic doctor with a leaning towards physical activity but is a distinct medical entity in itself. It has been defined by the Council of Europe Committee of

Ministers as 'the application of the art and science of medicine from a preventative and therapeutic point of view to the practice of sports and physical activities in order to utilize the opportunities accorded by sports for maintaining or improving health' (Resolution 73/27).

This book is intended to be a guide for the Accident Department and General Practice; it is hoped that it will be an aid in the diagnosis and treatment of such injuries which are mainly sports specific as well as defining the relationship of the more common injuries to athletic performance.

Chapter 2

Frequency and site of injury

Fortunately, serious sports injuries are rare. Minor cuts and bruises are an accepted part of any sporting endeavour but major injuries such as fractures, dislocations and complex lacerations are seen at relatively infrequent intervals. For example, in the author's experience of over 500 professional soccer matches there were two fractured tibiae, two major ligamentous injuries of the knee, one fracture-dislocation of the ankle, three facial injuries and four minor head injuries which required hospital admission. The overall injury rate (for minor and serious injuries) per hundred participants was 2·8.

However, personal reminiscences are no substitute for accurate records when assessing the frequency of a sports injury. Unfortunately most minor clubs do not compile details of sporting accidents and retrospective studies are usually unfruitful. The picture is also blurred because the frequency of a sports injury depends upon local or national popularity of each sport. *Table* 1 lists a study by Johansen (1955) in Oslo. As expected there is a predominance of skiing injuries (1784) and football injuries (1320) which reflected local popularity. *Table* 2 attempts to analyse the injury rate per hundred participants, each listed injury being serious enough to warrant the attention of the club doctor or trainer.

FREQUENCY PER HOURS PLAYED
In order to shed some light on the sports injury problem Weightman and Browne have carried out two prospective studies (1974, 1975). They assessed the injury rate per 10 000 hours of matchplay.

In the first study data were collected from 696 association football clubs and 117 rugby clubs. In all 6120 football accidents were reported and 1944 rugby accidents. Although the injury rate for rugby (30·5 per 10 000 hours) was lower than for soccer (36·5 per 10 000 hours)

Table 1. Injuries in Various Sports (Johansen, 1955) in One Year

Sport	Injuries
Skiing	1784
Football	1320
Gymnastics	622
Bathing and swimming	523
Handball	393
Skating	363
Tobogganing	279
Hockey and ice hockey	135
Wrestling	116
Boxing	100
Athletics	90
Cross-country running	57
Tennis	30
Other sports	245
Total	6057

Table 2. Sports Injury Rate per Hundred Participating (Muckle and Shepherdson, 1975)

Sport	Rate
Rugby	4·9
Skiing	4·9
Soccer	3·2
Gymnastics	2·9
Hockey	2·7
Judo	2·1
Rowing	2·1
Squash	2·0
Tennis	2·0
Boxing	1·7
Basketball	1·7

the former injuries were more serious as shown by the fact that hospital treatment was needed in 52·8 per cent of rugby injuries compared to 29·8 per cent of soccer injuries. Fractures and dislocations were twice as common in rugby and concussion more frequent. Allemandou (1976) reviewed 11 349 rugby injuries in France and found that 12·5 per cent of injuries happened in training and 46 per cent occurred when the players resumed playing after the summer break. The author also observed that the worst month for soccer injuries was August when the pre-season training and friendly matches were taking place; most of the injuries were of an intrinsic nature. Rugby injuries needed, on average, 12 days off play compared to 6 days in soccer.

In a further study Weightman and Browne (1975) surveyed the injury rate per hour in several sports (hockey, cricket, fencing, cycling, judo, rowing, boxing, sub-aquatic activities and swimming).

Table 3 gives the injury rate in each sport. Hockey comes third in the 'injury league', after soccer and rugby, with the rate for women marginally greater than for men (12·5 to 10·3 respectively). When water sports were studied rowing had a rate of 1·4, sub-aquatic activities 0·49 and swimming 0·3. Table 4 gives the incidence of injuries during sporting events involving children.

Eleven per cent of all injuries involve the head (La Cava, 1960). Boxing deserves special mention since an indirect brain injury is commonly produced by a blow to the chin, shearing stresses by blows to the side of the face and secondary injury as the head strikes the floor. However, in almost all series amateur boxing appears to be a relatively safe sport. Blonstein (1966) reported that in 4350 amateur boxing contests 136 serious injuries occurred, a 3 per cent incidence.

Table 3. Injuries per 10 000 Man-hours of Play (Weightman and Browne, 1975)

Soccer	36·5
Rugby	30·5
Hockey—women	12·5
Hockey—men	10·3
Fencing	4·2
Cricket	2·6
Judo	1·6
Cycling	1·56
Badminton	1·49
Rowing	1·4
Boxing	1·4
Sub-aquatic activities	0·49
Swimming	0·3

Table 4. Incidence of injuries by sport in children (Goldberg et al., 1979)

	%
AUGMENTED SPEED SPORTS	33·3
Skateboarding	15·7
Ice skating	5·9
Sledging	3·9
Skiing	3·9
Trampolining	2·0
Bicycling	2·0
COLLISION SPORTS	29·4
Football	27·5
Ice hockey	2·0
CONTACT SPORTS	27·5
Basketball	7·8
Volleyball	7·8
Soccer	5·9
Baseball	3·9
Field hockey	2·0
NON-CONTACT SPORTS	9·8
Tennis	3·9
Gymnastics	2·0
Swimming	2·0
Cross-country	2·0

Blonstein and Schmid (1974) showed in a preliminary report that the causes of death in ex-boxers were the same as in the normal population and the life-span between the two groups did not differ.

Barber (1973) showed that head injuries are frequent after horse-riding accidents. Of 154 serious accidents related to this sport in a 2-year period 101 patients were concussed and 7 had post-traumatic amnesia for more than 24 hours. An interesting point from this Oxford survey was that one hospital bed was permanently occupied by a horse-riding accident; two-thirds of the patients were teenagers and 109 were female. Only 36 patients were professionally employed in dealing with horses.

One of the commonest causes of serious sports injuries is skiing accidents. Throughout the world there has been an increase in the number of skiing injuries during the past decade, and published reports indicate that almost 500 000 people are injured each year. There are 225 000 fractures caused by this sport in the United States annually. Eriksson (1976) reported that 42 per cent of skiing injuries were found in the under-15 age group and the majority (75 per cent) occurred during downhill skiing; deficiencies in the slope were cited as the main cause of the accident. Skiing too fast and beyond the ability of the participant were also found to be common factors. Snow conditions affected the type of trauma produced. When edging conditions were poor (ice or extremely hard-packed snow) injuries to the upper extremities and trunk were more prevalent. With good edging conditions lower limb injuries were more frequent (Johnson et al., 1976). Overall, 72 per cent of skiing injuries affected the lower limb and in young skiers there was a high percentage of tibial fractures. The importance of good release bindings was emphasized by Eriksson (1976); the release group incurred fewer lower limb injuries (55 per cent) than the non-release group (80 per cent).

SUDDEN DEATH

Thankfully, deaths from sport are rare. Most fatalities occur with head and cervical spine injuries and are usually due to severe external forces such as being thrown from a vehicle or struck by a heavy ball or stick. Obviously certain speed sports (motor car and motor cycle racing) and airborne pursuits (hang-gliding and ordinary gliding) have an inherent danger which is difficult to eliminate. Swimming, which features in *Table 3* as a safe pursuit, is associated with a high mortality from drowning due to the large number of participants. Blonstein (1966) reported no deaths in amateur boxing over a 7-year period during which 60 000 senior amateur boxers participated annually.

Shephard (1974) has reviewed the literature on sudden death during exercise and points out that unaccustomed physical activity, especially in middle age, may precipitate ventricular fibrillation and myocardial infarction. In a full review of the subject Shephard quotes an incidence of 8 attacks of ventricular fibrillation per 50 000 gym-hours.

SITE OF INJURY

Fig. 1 shows the sites of injury in participants of all sports. However, *Fig.* 2 is based on the work of Weightman and Browne (1975) and breaks down the injuries into various sports.

Head and facial injuries are not uncommon; 30 per cent of all rugby injuries are to these areas, most being simple cuts and bruises; teeth were commonly displaced and jaw injuries accounted for 28·8 per cent. In hockey 33 per cent of all injuries were to the head and face and lacerations from broken spectacles were not infrequent. In cricket about one-quarter of the total injuries were head and facial; concussion from a fast delivery was not uncommon.

Shoulder injuries are frequent in rugby and American football with 'arm tackling' in the latter producing hyperextension of the abducted arm thus predisposing to shoulder dislocations. Acromioclavicular injuries were fairly frequent in soccer, American football and judo. Half of the injuries in fencing were to the upper limbs but were mostly cuts and bruises. Of all injuries found in judo one-third were to the upper limbs, where fractures and dislocations were not infrequent. One-quarter of serious injuries in hurling were fractures of the fingers.

As could be expected, the lower limbs suffer a fairly large proportion of the total injuries whatever sport is studied. Sixty-five per cent of all soccer injuries and 30 per cent of rugby injuries are to these areas. Soccer players regularly sustain cuts and bruises to the tibial

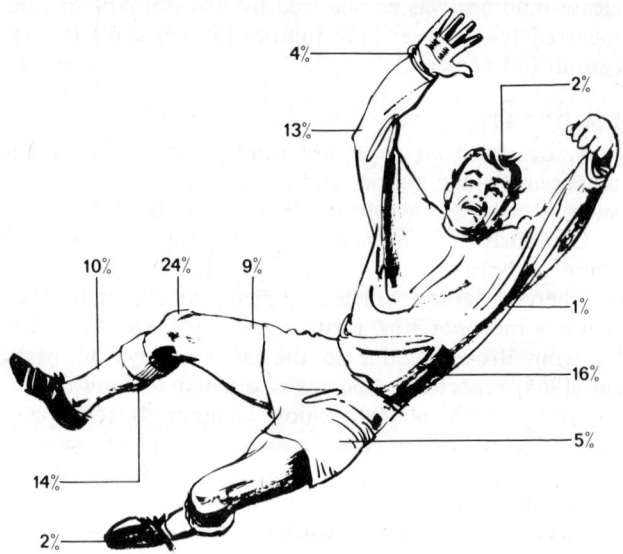

Fig. 1. The site of injury; the percentages represent all sports.

FREQUENCY AND SITE OF INJURY

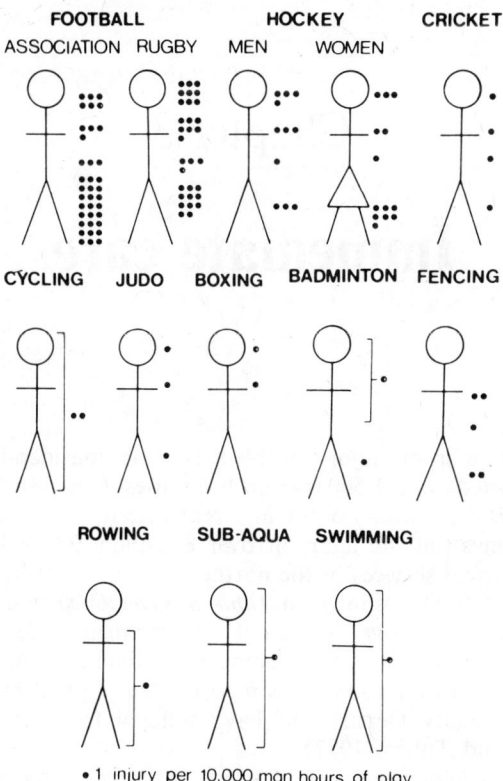

Fig. 2. Injuries in various sports (Weightman and Browne, 1975).

region, thigh and ankle. More than 50 per cent of hockey injuries, 80 per cent in rowing and 63 per cent in badminton were to the legs with pulled muscles, meniscal injuries and ankle strains predominating. The knee menisci and ligaments, and the ankle ligaments suffer in many sports including skiing, squash, American football, soccer, rugby, basketball, volleyball, high jumping, long jumping, tennis, cross-country running and figure skating.

Thus the data in this chapter indicate that although sports injuries cover a very broad spectrum of body trauma, the chances of a serious injury per hours played is quite low.

Chapter 3

Immediate care

The size of the sports injury problem is quite considerable—in 1963 Morris reported that 1 500 000 such injuries (sufficiently severe to keep the person off work) occur in Great Britain each year and more recent estimates put the figure at over 2 million. The estimated load upon the hospital services in the northern area studied by Weightman and Browne (1975) is shown in *Table 5*. Over 6000 injuries required medical attention in the Accident Department and these are only a small percentage of the total needing immediate care on the field of play or in the dressing room. It is reported that 7 per cent of all attenders at a Casualty Department have suffered from a sports injury (Crompton and Tubbs, 1977).

One of the unique features of sports medicine is the fact that the doctor is often present at the moment of injury and is thus responsible for some of the immediate care (or first aid).

Table 5. Sports Injuries treated in Hospital in One Year (Weightman and Browne, 1975)

Injury	Number	Percentage
Cuts and bruises	2348	35·9
Fractures and dislocations	2315	35·4
Sprains, soft-tissue injuries	1405	21·5
Concussion	283	4·3
Soft-tissue swelling and blisters	143	2·2
Broken teeth	37	0·6
Other	3	0·05
Total	6534	

FIRST AID FACILITIES

The importance of first aid facilities has been emphasized in many reports (including Weightman and Browne, 1975; Muckle, 1976). Although it is ideal to have first aid facilities for all players many minor clubs fail in this respect. It has been shown that only 74 per cent of soccer clubs, 46 per cent of rugby clubs, 43 per cent of boxing clubs, 32 per cent of hockey clubs and 5 per cent of rowing clubs have first aid facilities (Weightman and Browne, 1975).

Before any event the medical adviser must ensure that the first aid equipment is in order. Stretchers, pneumatic splints, bandages, sutures, etc. should be readily available in a treatment room which should be clean, warm and well-illuminated. The basic medical equipment is listed in *Table 6*.

Table 6. Medical Equipment required in the First Aid Treatment of Athletes (Muckle and Shepherdson, 1975)

Stretcher, splints, wooden board or support for spinal injuries
A supply of crêpe and cotton bandages, including a triangular bandage
Sterile dressings of various sizes, cotton-wool, tulle gras, Elastoplast and other adhesive plasters
Adhesive felt padding. Tubigrip (for knee and ankle). Adhesive sponge rubber
Mild antiseptic solutions
A ready supply of warm water, cold ice pack (ice cubes or a proprietary brand), towels, footbaths, wax hand-baths
Eye bath. Chloramphenicol drops, small glass rod, fluorescein
Sterile water
Dextrose–saline solutions, intravenous giving sets plus needles
Dumb-bell or Steristrip sutures, steritape
Black silk sutures, nylon sutures (1–6/0), dexon, needles, forceps, scissors, as a suture pack. Scalpels and supply of blades
Local anaesthetics, including a long-acting variety
Syringes and needles of various sizes
Adrenaline for nose bleeds, in solution. Nasal drops
Local steroids. Local anaesthetic sprays
Antibiotics. Anti-inflammatory agents. Antidiarrhoeal medicine
Antibiotic skin sprays, 'plastic' covering sprays. Steroid creams
Tetanus toxoid
Hypnotics (Mogadon). Antihistamines
Petroleum jelly, olive oil, smelling salts, antifungal powder and ointment
Chiropody kit with disposable scalpels
Liquid glucose, glucose tablets
Talcum powder, shampoos, soaps
Embrocation. Xylocaine ointment
Clinical thermometer, stethoscope, ophthalmoscope, auriscope, sphygmomanometer

---

The proximity of an Accident Service will determine the necessity for emergency packs for cardiac and thoracic resuscitation, e.g. intercostal drainage sets, ECG machines. This particularly applies to sporting events involving high speeds.

THE AVOIDANCE OF INJURY

It is pertinent to look at the injury problem before it begins. The avoidance of injury requires a correct warming-up period. The athlete should spend approximately 20 minutes stretching key muscle groups while exercising on the track or on a firm but pliable surface such as thick all-purpose carpeting over a wooden gym floor.

Players suffering from illnesses such as boils, tonsillitis, heavy colds, glandular fever, etc. should not participate because they are more liable to injury through fatigue as well as the disease process itself. The author has seen a ruptured spleen in a soccer player suffering from glandular fever who received a minor abdominal blow, and torn hamstrings have been observed beneath a large carbuncle of the thigh. Two simple but golden rules are that players should not train before being fully fit after illness or injury, and they should never use faulty or inadequate equipment.

Training before a match should be thorough with an emphasis both on skill and endurance because a fatigued player is more prone to cause or suffer an injury, e.g. a mistimed tackle in soccer can put both players at risk.

PRINCIPLES OF IMMEDIATE TREATMENT

The following general principles apply—be prepared for the unexpected, keep calm and use common sense.

Prompt treatment prevents further damage which is caused in two ways. First, forces applied across the injured area continue to tear or stretch the retaining structures. Second, more blood and oedema are forced into the injured tissues thus increasing pain, swelling and subsequent fibrosis. Many players will attempt to persevere for a short period after injury before abandoning the event. The medical adviser should forbid this resumption having previously made it quite clear to the club management and captain that such medical decisions are the prerogative of the doctor and not the player concerned.

If there is any doubt as to the seriousness of the injury the player can be carried off on a stretcher or the injured limb supported by splints; a more diligent examination is made in the dressing room or Casualty Department.

Emergency Treatment

Fig. 3 gives the emergency assessment of an injured person; certain points need emphasis. In an unconscious player the teeth should be inspected to make sure that loose fragments have not been inhaled, and foreign bodies, e.g. chewing gum, are removed from the mouth. The pupils are rapidly inspected and their reaction to light noted.

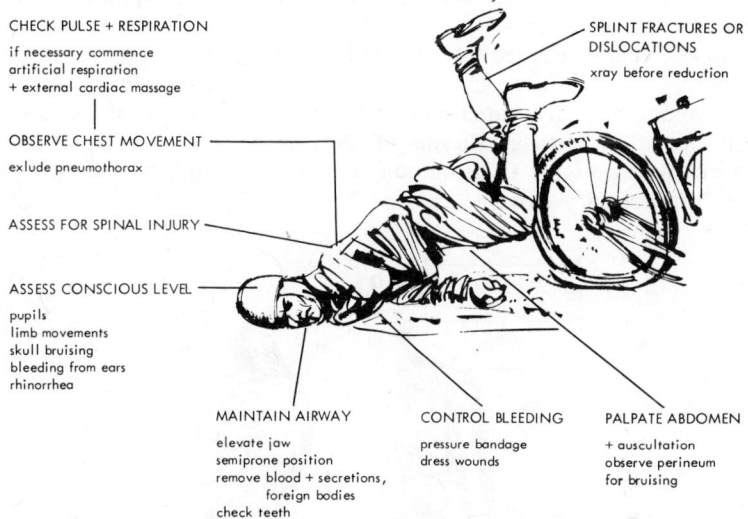

Fig. 3. Emergency treatment in an injured sportsman.

Scalp wounds are sought, eye and limb movements watched, and the spine examined swiftly for injury. Clothes can be cut off the injured area to avoid unnecessary movement. Splints should be gently and quickly applied, recalling the maxim 'splint them where they lie'. If a spinal injury is suspected the player must be transported on a firm stretcher with the head immobilized between rolled blankets. Even if a joint dislocation is believed to have occurred there should be no attempt at immediate reduction until a radiograph has excluded a concurrent fracture, e.g. the humeral head in a dislocated shoulder or the trochlea in a dislocated elbow.

Assessment of Nerve and Vascular Damage

The main areas where nerves are damaged in sporting injuries are given in *Fig.* 4. Nerve concussion (neuropraxia) is common after kicks and blows to the limbs especially as a form of 'dead leg' following a posterior thigh blow. The numb feeling usually subsides in a few hours. Intrathecal rupture of the nerve fibres (axonotmesis) occurs with a severe stretching injury or even a dislocation (e.g. axillary nerve damage with a shoulder dislocation) and may take several weeks to recover. However, recovery is often complete. Nerve severance (neurotmesis) is commonly found with a laceration or fracture, especially when there is gross displacement of jagged bone ends. Operative intervention is required, the best results following repair with an operating microscope.

Absent pulses, reduced warmth, pallor and numbness indicate vascular injury which can be due to direct rupture, pressure from increasing swelling or a dislocated bone, intimal tears, bruising of the vessel wall and arterial spasm. Bleeding from external surfaces can be controlled by a pressure dressing coupled with splinting of the limb to avoid unnecessary movement.

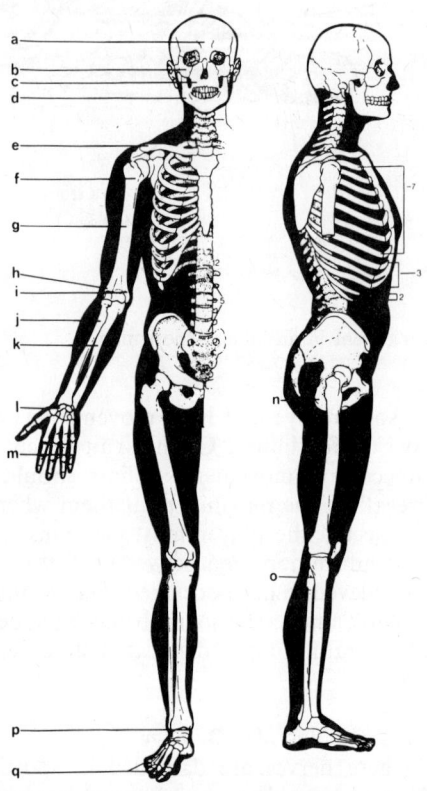

Fig. 4. Principal areas of nerve damage. **a**, Supraorbital in lacerations; **b**, Infraorbital in zygomatic fractures; **c + d**, Dental nerves in maxilla and mandibular fractures; **e**, Brachial plexus in clavicular and traction injuries; **f**, Axillary nerve in shoulder dislocations; **g**, Radial nerve in humeral fractures; **h**, Median nerve in elbow injuries; **i**, Ulnar nerve in elbow dislocations; **j**, Posterior interosseous with upper radial fractures or dislocations; **k**, Anterior interosseous with forearm injuries; **l**, Median nerve with carpal dislocations; **m**, Digital nerves with finger injuries; **n**, Sciatic nerve with pelvic dislocations or hip injuries; **o**, Lateral popliteal nerve with fibular fractures; **p**, Anterior or posterior tibial nerve injury with tibial fractures; **q**, digital nerves with foot injuries.

Assessment of Head and Spinal Injuries

It is a golden rule that all sportsmen having been unconscious should stop playing; to resume activity with its tenfold increase in blood flow may aggravate or precipitate intracranial bleeding. The player is taken to hospital for skull radiographs and many Casualty Departments wisely admit the patient for a 24-hour period of observation.

The single most important observation is an accurate and periodically recorded assessment of the conscious level. When the pupils dilate as a result of rising intracranial pressure, the pupil on the side of the lesion dilates first. Immediate ophthalmoscopic examination may reveal vitreous or fundal haemorrhages, but frank papilloedema is rarely seen in the first few hours after injury. The limbs are observed for both spontaneous and reflex movement although the tendon reflexes may be of little value in the initial assessment. Hemiparesis or hemiplegia may be caused by a compressing intracranial lesion, cerebral laceration or contusion; while compression of the midbrain against the free edge of the tentorium may produce false localizing signs. Severe weakness in one upper limb may indicate a brachial plexus lesion; bilateral limb weakness and sensory impairment may be due to spinal trauma.

Scalp wounds should not be probed and no attempt should be made to remove tissue because if a piece of skull bone has been driven into a dural sinus or cortical vein its removal may result in brisk bleeding. The scalp wound is simply covered with a sterile dressing until full casualty facilities are on hand. The external auditory meatuses are examined for blood, which may indicate a fractured base of skull, a torn pinna, meatal canal or tympanic membrane. Epistaxis is common, but rhinorrhoea is proof of an open paranasal sinus fracture with a tear of the dura mater. Malar, maxillary and mandibular fractures can be detected clinically by defects of occlusion, malalignment and crepitus.

Garfield (1973) has pointed out that unless there is gross neurological deficit the initial assessment of spinal damage, including cord involvement, is difficult. Observation of the spinal contour on the field of play is best made by rolling the player on to the side while maintaining gentle head traction. The detection of a cervical fracture or fracture-dislocation can be assumed from cervical pain, muscle spasm, difficulty in moving the head and neurological changes in the upper limbs. If such an injury is suspected the neck is immobilized with rolled blankets, a pair of sandbags or an orthopaedic collar. A small step or kyphos in the thoracic region may indicate vertebral injury. Pain and tenderness may be slight with crush fractures of the lumbar spine, or pain may be referred to the buttocks and legs. In all cases of suspected spinal injury the athlete is transferred in the neutral position on a firm stretcher or boards with gentle traction on the head in the case of high spinal damage.

Soft-tissue Injury
The immediate treatment is discussed in Chapter 4.

It is worth pointing out that the immediate care of the injured sportsman is the first stage of rehabilitation and an essential period of treatment. The unique opportunity of the sports medicine doctor to be present at the event or on the field of play should mean that the initial therapy (designed to safeguard life and prevent further damage) is correctly and swiftly carried out.

Chapter 4

Soft-tissue injuries—acute

IMMEDIATE CARE
Soft-tissue injuries may occur on their own or in association with a fracture or dislocation; in the latter event they are often overlooked. Immediately after injury (on the field of play) the damage area is rested in a sling, collar and cuff, crêpe-and-wool support or a splint; in serious cases a stretcher is provided. Once the player is in the treatment room a careful clinical assessment is made and therapy commenced.

Injuries to muscles, tendons, ligaments, capsules, fascia and skin readily bleed and tissue fluid rapidly accumulates. Immediate attention is directed towards limiting or preventing these complications as well as arresting further soft-tissue damage (*Fig.* 5).

The régime is recalled by the ICE rule—ice, compression and elevation. A cold compress is applied to the elevated limb for 20–60 minutes

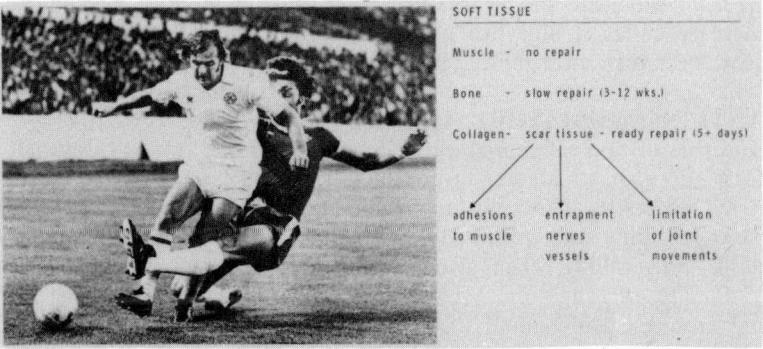

Fig. 5. The variation in response to injury by the soft tissues must be taken into account when planning treatment and rehabilitation. (*Photograph by M. Rous, Oxford.*)

depending on the amount of swelling. A proprietary solution can be used for cooling, but the simplest method is to place ice cubes in a thick towel or an iced solution in a rubber bottle and mould the cold compress around the injured area. Ice should never be applied directly to the skin or a burn may result. The injured area is rested in a crêpe-and-wool support or plaster for 48 hours when an inspection can be carried out. Then ligament and tendon injuries should show signs of resolution while muscle injuries can be graded into intermuscular and intramuscular. Small effusions are treated conservatively but large effusions, especially haemarthroses, should be aspirated and reaspirated if they reaccumulate. Otherwise this is the period of non-therapy. It is worth recalling that recent injuries cannot be run off; heated away; massaged, stretched or manipulated away; electrically stimulated or injected away. Any meddlesome activity within the first 24–48 hours will only make the swelling worse, delay resolution and increase fibrosis.

BIOCHEMISTRY OF SOFT-TISSUE TRAUMA

Capillary haemorrhage and oedema, synovial swelling and lysosomal disruption accompany trauma to soft tissues, and at the same time local chemicals are released and play a part in the pathological processes. These chemical agents, e.g. histamine, serotonin, bradykinin and various polypeptides, have for many years been thought to be the main instigators of the local soft-tissue response to injury. However, recent interest has centred around the possible role of prostaglandins released by non-specific tissue damage. Prostaglandins E_1 and E_2 are involved in pain production, potentiation and increased vascular permeability, thus causing persistent oedema and late fibrosis. In addition, small amounts of prostaglandin E compounds, if allowed to persist at the site of injury, can render the area painful for several weeks (Andersen and Ramwell, 1974). Prostaglandins E_1 and $F_{1\alpha}$ increase collagen biosynthesis and may be responsible for excessive scar formation after injury (Blumenkrantz and Søndergaard, 1972).

ANTI-INFLAMMATORY AGENTS

The role of anti-inflammatory agents in soft-tissue trauma, especially their effects on prostaglandin production and release, has been investigated (Muckle, 1974). In a double-blind trial ibuprofen (Brufen) 1200 mg daily and aspirin 3 g daily (*Fig.* 6) were shown to reduce pain and swelling when given immediately after injury. This study and a later investigation (Muckle, 1977) using flurbiprofen were carried out amongst professional soccer players; immediately after injury the player received the standard ICE therapy plus a 5-day supply of an anti-inflammatory compound. All injuries requiring such therapies as joint aspiration, ultrasound, manipulation, etc. were excluded from these

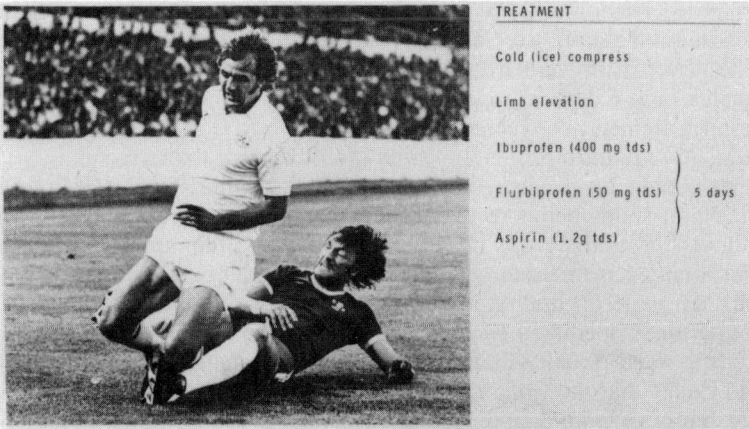

Fig. 6. Initial treatment of soft-tissue injuries (Muckle, 1974; 1976). (*Photograph by M. Rous, Oxford.*)

trials in order to assess the value of the anti-inflammatory agents. The ibuprofen-treated group (30 players) had a greater pain relief and returned to training after 3·8 days compared to 6·6 days with the aspirin group (30 players). These differences were significant. An important feature was the initial loading dose of ibuprofen (2 tab or 800 mg) within hours (sometimes minutes) of injury. More recent studies have indicated an ibuprofen dosage of up to 2400 mg daily for 5 days.

However, further trials were undertaken to answer certain fundamental questions. The first question was whether these trials could show that anti-inflammatory agents had an effect in sports injuries. A comparison of indomethacin (150 mg daily) and placebo in professional footballers showed no statistical difference (only 15 players in each group) when pain relief and resumption of training were studied (Huskisson et al., 1973). However, these results are contrary to other investigations which have found a beneficial action of indomethacin in musculoskeletal disorders (Leclerc and Autissier, 1969). A further study (Valtonen and Busson, 1978) showed no difference between ibuprofen 1200 mg daily and indomethacin 75 mg daily in 60 cases of soft tissue disorders. Both were effective but indomethacin had slightly more side-effects, notably gastric upset. In other series both benorylate tablets and naproxen 250 mg t.d.s. have been found to be effective in sports injuries. The second important question to be asked is whether anti-inflammatory tablets have a negative effect, i.e. retard healing and thus predispose to recurrence. For example, one could argue that drug A had no effect, but appeared better than B because the latter drug retarded healing and recovery. To answer this question aspirin given 3 g and 3·6 g daily were compared (Muckle, 1980b). The players given the larger dose trained at 4·2 days, compared to 6·6 days, and were match fit at 6 days, compared to 9·5 days. Thus the beneficial effects of aspirin seemed to be related to dosage in a positive manner. In the same trial 150 mg flurbiprofen appeared more effective than aspirin.

It should be recalled that most soft-tissue injuries are self-limiting and that spontaneous recovery occurs irrespective of treatment. In the above studies there was no reported increase in the number of players sustaining a recurrence of injury because healing was incomplete. But further experimental studies are required to ensure that collagen biosynthesis mediated by prostaglandins (F 2α) is not being affected.

In general practice many sports injuries present days later. There is no doubt that anti-inflammatory agents work best when given within 24 hours of injury, and animal experiments support this conclusion (Adams, 1980). Even so, results from two surveys in sports clinics have shown that ibuprofen 1600 mg daily is effective when given within a few days of injury (Bourne and Bentley, 1980; Crane, Gibson and Busson, 1980).

But in chronic injuries such as groin strain, Achilles tendinitis and tennis elbow, anti-inflammatory agents do not seem to confer any benefit other than having an analgesic action.

PROPHYLAXIS

In theory, these drugs could be given before an event to prevent the effects of injury, e.g. in boxing or karate. However, phenylbutazone has been banned in horse racing and the author at present believes that the prophylactic use of anti-inflammatory agents is not justified.

There are various reasons. Drugs may artificially augment performance by preventing injury, mask an injury so that a further, and more serious, injury occurs (e.g. partial to complete tearing of a ligament), cause side-effects in patients and pave the way for other and potentially more dangerous drugs (such as the butazones, etc.) to be given regularly.

What are the conclusions? Anti-inflammatory agents appear to accelerate the rate of recovery in sports injuries when given early. This is important to men and women in sport who are keen to regain match-fitness as rapidly as possible. The availability of safe, simple therapy compatible with this aim is important to this group.

Thus anti-inflammatory agents have a part to play in the immediate treatment of a soft-tissue injury, supplementing other, more traditional methods of rest, elevation, strapping and plaster-of-Paris immobilization. The relative paucity of side-effects in fit persons over a short course of 5-7 days makes one of the non-steroidal anti-inflammatory agents the drug of choice.

ENZYME PREPARATIONS

Hyaluronidase is useful in acute soft-tissue injuries especially when hydrocortisone or other steroids have been given locally (such as in tenosynovitis of the wrist). However, the use of oral enzyme preparations is hindered by their vulnerability to gastric acidity although many are enteric coated. Although undoubtedly popular, objective scientific evidence regarding the usefulness of oral enzymes in soft-tissue trauma is still difficult to find, indeed in one double-blind trial of chymotrypsin plus trypsin in ankle sprains no benefit was found over placebo (Craig, 1975).

Local applications of heparinoid substance, methyl salicylate liniment (oil of wintergreen), turpentine liniment, white liniment and cooling sprays have a soothing effect on the skin, but there is little convincing evidence to support their efficacy in the treatment of soft-tissue injuries, and most are of historical interest only.

PHYSICAL THERAPY

After a 48-hour rest period, when the biochemical tide has begun to subside with the corresponding reduction in pain and swelling, the crucially important phase of muscle and joint facilitation begins. In severe injuries the injured limb may have to be rested for several days, but after 48 hours static (isometric) exercises commence under supervision. Once the athlete has been encouraged to master these exercises then he can carry them out on his own on a strict time schedule, e.g. 5 minutes of exercises every hour. Such exercises aid remodelling of the newly produced scar tissue, help to prevent adhesions and reduce oedema. They also facilitate neurosensory feedback from muscles, tendons and ligaments—ultimately helping to restore full proprioception, power and balance. Increased muscle power can also control any temporary ligamentous instability as well as taking the joint through a full range of movement, thus aiding hyaline cartilage nutrition.

This progression from passive to active joint movements requires care, patience and strict supervision. Each exercise should be fully mastered and be relatively painless before embarking on another part of the programme. Ice facilitation is extremely useful both by its analgesic action and also in controlling swelling. However, contrast-bathing within 48 hours of injury is not recommended because the 'heat factor' may potentiate oedema.

In the U.S.A. an isokinetic dynamometer (such as the Cybex II) is used by many sporting organizations as part of the rehabilitation programme. Such apparatus allows observations and quantifications of the basic muscle strength through a range of motion, explosive power and endurance. Print-out data on these specific aspects is useful in injury evaluation, measuring rehabilitation progress and for screening individuals for injury prevention programmes. The expense of such instrumentation (approximately $10 000) puts it beyond most sporting organisations.

However, there is no substitute for the skill and encouragement of a trained supervisor during the transition from passive to active exercises, the judicious use of weights, and the return to vigorous field activity.

Electrical apparatus holds a certain 'mystique' for athletes. Ultrasound speeds tissue regeneration in experimental animals and is said to stimulate the secretion of collagen precursors in the human fibroblast. However, its precise effect in the healing process after soft-tissue injuries has not been fully evaluated, although it is often effective in tenosynovitis, ligamentous strain and certain enthesiopathies, such as tennis elbow or plantar fasciitis. Short-wave diathermy and radiant heat are useful adjuncts to the exercise programme when local swelling has begun to subside. They not only give a feeling of well-being but have a counter-irritant effect on the skin, thus decreasing or blocking painful stimuli in the complex neurological pathways of the spinal cord (the gate-effect).

LIGAMENT INJURY
These are divided into *sprain*, *partial tear* and *complete tear*. It is not unusual to tear one side of a joint and crush the other. A dislocation is usually accompanied by major ligamentous damage.

Sprain
This is diagnosed by localized tenderness and restricted movement without much oedema or joint swelling, and no abnormal joint mobility is found. Usually responds to 3–14 days' immobilization with strapping or crêpe-and-wool.

Partial Tear
The above signs are more severe and joint swelling is present. However, no abnormal joint mobility occurs. If necessary, the joint is aspirated to relieve haemarthrosis and plaster immobilization instituted for 3 weeks.

Complete Tear
Excessive mobility, severe pain and major haemarthrosis indicate the serious nature of the injury. Stress radiographs or an arthrogram can be used to reach a diagnosis, but the severity of symptoms usually necessitates a surgical exploration to ascertain the extent of damage and to undertake repair. A plaster is applied for 4–6 weeks.

Special Ligamentous Injuries

Rotator cuff tears will be reviewed in Chapter 10; knee and ankle ligamentous injuries are described in Chapters 8 and 9 respectively.

Sprains of the *medial ligament of elbow* are not uncommon in javelin throwers with a faulty 'round-arm' action (Miller, 1960), whereas the expert thrower may develop olecranon and triceps lesions. Elbow injuries in throwers are typically of the whiplash type and are due to hyperextension at the elbow joint (*Fig.* 7), as a result of which the olecranon impinges on the floor of its fossa. In some cases a fracture may result or a severe strain of the anterior capsule. Loose bodies and small ossicles (resembling osteochondritis dissecans) may be found in the olecranon fossa. Treatment is rest, plaster for 2–3 weeks, alteration in style or removal of loose bodies and osteophytes.

Severe sprains and partial tears of the *ligaments of the fingers*, especially the interphalangeal ligaments, are found in participants of rugby, wrestling, skiing and similar sports (Flatt, 1969). The *ulnar collateral ligament of the thumb* may be torn from its attachment at the base of the proximal phalanx and can be prevented from uniting by the interposition of the abductor aponeurosis. Surgical repair is required to give a stable joint.

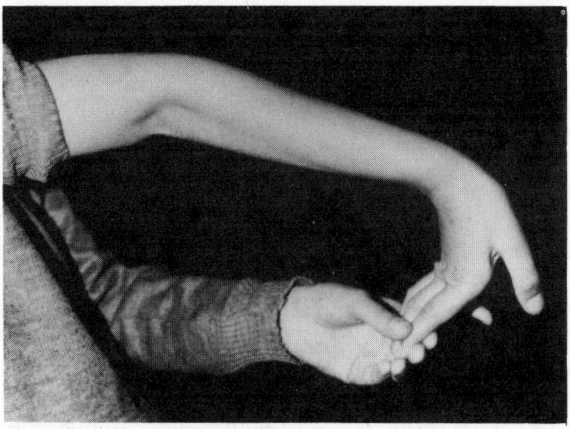

Fig. 7. Familial joint hypermobility in a young gymnast. Such mobility may be associated with valgus ankles and 'apparent' flat feet; and an increased liability to ligamentous injury and osteoarthrosis in later life.

ACUTE TENDON INJURY

These are divided into *partial* and *complete*.

In young people muscles are ruptured more than tendons; in older persons the reverse is true. A tendon may rupture either during normal activity or during abnormal physical stress. The avulsion of a tendon

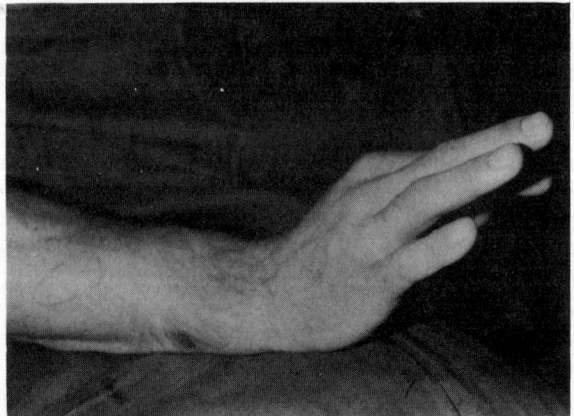

Fig. 8. Isolated rupture of the extensor indices following a blow from a squash racket (area outlined).

from its insertion into bone is almost always traumatic (*Fig.* 8), as is a rupture at the musculotendinous junction. Rupture occurs within a tendon only if it is abnormal, either from intrinsic degeneration or from wearing and fraying from friction. The best treatment of a fresh rupture of a large or important tendon is accurate apposition of its ends without tension until healing is complete. Severely frayed or degenerate parts should always be excised; in some instances the defect can be bridged with a free tendon graft but in other cases a tendon transfer is best.

Bicipital tendinitis (golfer's, baseball or tennis shoulder) may be difficult to differentiate from partial tears of the long head of biceps. Both conditions respond to rest, analgesics and gentle exercises. Although local steroids can be used in the former there is the danger of converting a partial into a complete tear; thus it is better to withhold steroids. Rarely the humeral insertion of pectoralis major may be torn in a throwing event and simulate a rupture of the long head of biceps (Chapter 10). Surgical repair is carried out.

The tendon of biceps may be displaced from the intertubercular groove; this can be verified by getting the athlete to hold a 4 kg dumbbell in each hand with the limb extended and externally rotated above the head. When the arm is lowered to 90–110° or so an audible snap and sharp pain are found and the examining fingers may feel the tendon displaced. If the symptoms are disabling a fascial repair of the transverse humeral ligament is performed or the long head can be anchored in the intertubercular groove (Chapter 10).

Tears of the triceps occur in throwing, especially the javelin (*Fig.* 9). Direct suture with plaster-of-Paris for 3 weeks in extension is recom-

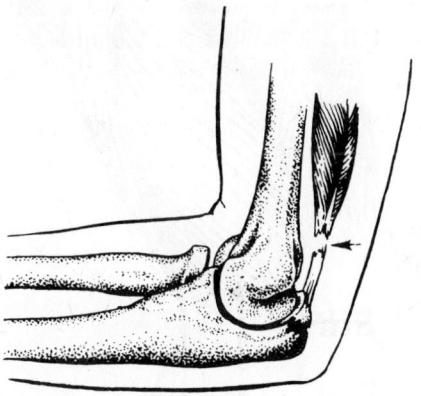

Fig. 9. Rupture of the triceps tendon and avulsion fracture of the olecranon.

mended, with an avulsion fracture a figure-of-8 tension band wiring is performed.

TENOSYNOVITIS OF THE WRIST
Common in racket players and oarsmen it responds to local steroids, hyaluronidase, anti-inflammatory agents and strapping. Two weeks later sport can begin; refractory cases require 2–4 weeks in plaster.

RUPTURE OF THE QUADRICEPS AND PATELLAR TENDONS
The quadriceps tendon usually ruptures transversely just proximal to the patella. The rupture should be repaired within 48 hours since the best results follow early surgery. Reinforcing sutures are desirable since the tear may occur through an area of degeneration. Direct repair and McLaughlin techniques (1947) are depicted (*Fig.* 10).

Rupture of the patellar tendon usually occurs at the inferior border of the patella; the McLaughlin repair (1947) can be carried out (*Fig.* 10*b*).

After the above operations a plaster cylinder with non-weight-bearing is used for 3 weeks with the knee in extension. Then the plaster is changed to a long leg plaster which is worn for a further 3 weeks; partial weight-bearing can be allowed during this period. Walking independently is commenced at 6 weeks, with a knee brace, if necessary. After 8 weeks' full extension and at least 50° of flexion should be possible, but maximum flexion may take 6–12 months. Sport is resumed once full knee movements have been regained.

RUPTURE OF THE PLANTARIS OR GASTROCNEMIUS
Rarely the fine tendon of plantaris may rupture as it passes down the

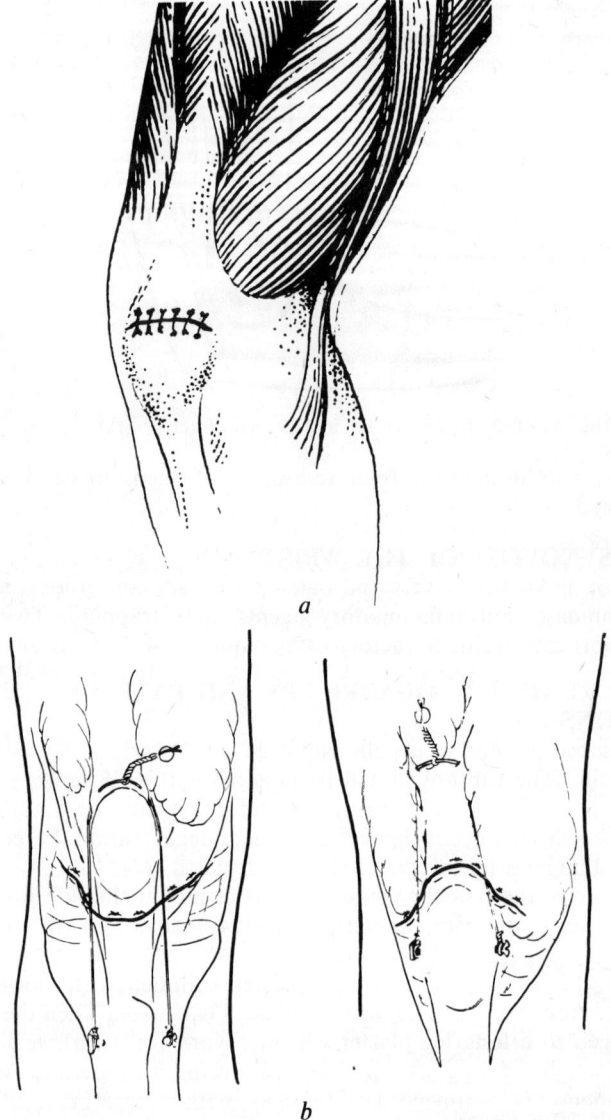

Fig. 10. Operations for rupture of the extensor mechanism of the knee. *a*, Avulsion of the superior pole of the patella treated by direct suture. Wire can be used but causes irritation and is associated with an increased risk of infection. At surgery the hyaline cartilage is inspected for damage. Perfect congruity of bone and cartilage must be obtained; otherwise it is better to excise the smaller fragment or, in severe cases, the patella. *b*, McLaughlin technique for both patellar tendon (*left*) and quadriceps tendon (*right*) (McLaughlin, 1947).

medial aspect of the Achilles tendon (tennis leg). However, the plantaris tendon rupture is often overdiagnosed. Generally this robust structure remains intact even in the presence of an Achilles tendon tear. One surgical procedure utilizes the plantaris tendon for repair (*see later*). The symptoms may mimic a partial tear of the Achilles tendon, but palpation of the latter does not reveal local tenderness and the athlete is able to stand comfortably on the toes. No therapy is required other than strapping and analgesics. Sport can begin in 2–3 weeks.

Occasionally the Achilles tendon tears at the musculotendinous junction, or the medial or lateral head of gastrocnemius may be partially ruptured. Strapping usually suffices but sometimes a full leg plaster is required if symptoms are slow in resolving or are initially severe. The plaster-of-Paris is applied for 3–6 weeks with the foot in the plantigrade position as for Achilles tendon rupture. However, since the gastrocnemius muscle arises from the femoral condyles a full leg plaster must be used. Sometimes, scarring on the deep surface of gastrocnemius leads to adhesions to the underlying soleus, with pain or discomfort on running and jumping. A similar problem may follow an undisplaced tibial fracture when there has been excessive bleeding in the calf.

TENOSYNOVITIS OF THE ANKLE
Repeated kicking in soccer can produce a tenosynovitis chiefly affecting the dorsiflexors of the toes. It responds to local steroids and strapping for 3–7 days. Often in professional footballers there are numerous capsular osteophytes which may cause ankle pain due to impingement or fracture. This pain may be misdiagnosed as tenosynovitis of the ankle.

STRAINS OF THE TIBIALIS POSTERIOR AND PERONEI
Any contact sport with body checking may cause strains of the above tendons and swelling and bruising is localized to the affected tendon sheaths. The best treatment is firm strapping or a plaster for 2 weeks. Sometimes excessive scarring results in nerve entrapment and tethering of the tendons. Surgical release may be needed under these circumstances. It is also worth noting that an ankle haemarthrosis may escape through a torn ligament and into the peroneal sheath.

SNAPPING TENDONS
These are of nuisance value only; in the hip a fascial band may slip over the greater trochanter; snapping shoulder may be caused by the long head of biceps displacing in the sulcus or by the supraspinatus syndrome; snapping scapula may be due to an exostosis on the thoracic cage or the body of the scapula itself; snapping knee may be due to an

exostosis on the medial aspect of the tibia which impinges on the pes anserinus during flexion and extension movements, occasionally the knee feels locked and a small bruise may appear on the inner aspect of the knee.

Treatment
The above lesions only require surgery if they become painful or disabling; in the case of the knee lesion described the exostosis is removed.

DISPLACEMENT OF THE PERONEAL TENDONS
The tendons are displaced from their normal position on the posterior surface of the lateral malleolus and lie obliquely over the lateral third of the distal surface of the fibula; since their fulcrum of pull is lost, their mechanical efficiency is impaired. This is not an uncommon injury in professional sportsmen, especially in contact sports such as rugger and soccer. It is simply diagnosed, the tendons often making audible clicks as they sublux. They are easily felt on the surface of the lateral malleolus.

Treatment
The groove is deepened and once the tendons have been replaced a repair or reconstruction of the superior retinaculum (*Fig.* 11) is carried

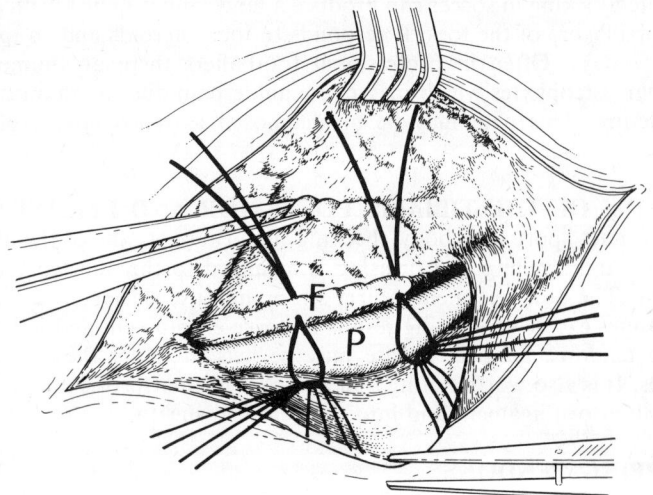

Fig. 11. An operation for displacement of peroneal tendons. The sutures in the superior retinaculum (bottom) are pulled through drill holes in the fibula (F) by means of guide sutures. P indicates the peroneal tendons. When the retinaculum is deficient a flap of periosteum can be taken from the fibula or the tendon of plantaris used (After Alm et al., 1975).

out. Conservative treatment is disappointing (Eckert and Davies, 1976). A plaster cast at 90° with eversion at the ankle is worn for 4 weeks. In refractory cases more complex surgical procedures are performed.

RUPTURE OF THE ACHILLES TENDON
The Achilles tendon may rupture close to the musculotendinous junction or near its insertion into the calcaneus. Areas of collagen degeneration may be found in the tendon bundles (*Fig.* 12).

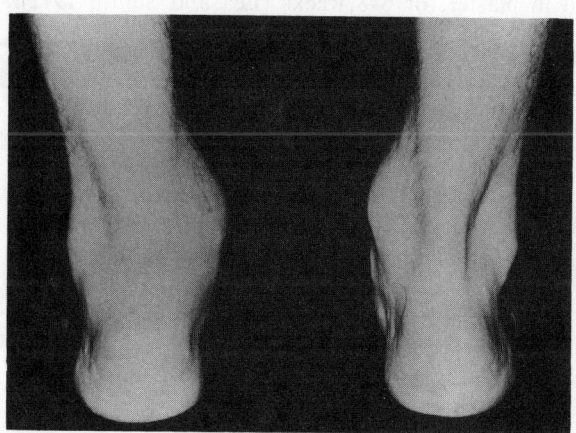

Fig. 12. Rupture of the left Achilles tendon after tennis.

Diagnosis
There is a sudden onset of pain in the heel region or calf and the player may feel he has been struck or tackled from behind. There is an inability to stand on tiptoe, and plantar flexion is weak and not accompanied by tautening of the tendon. A gap is usually palpable 5 cm or so above the heel, and squeezing the calf does not produce plantar flexion. Local steroid injections predispose to rupture.

Partial tears may simply present as mild swelling around the lower part of the Achilles tendon with local tenderness and foot movements are normal. Often partial tears are diagnosed as Achilles tendinitis.

When a complete tear is not seen for 24–48 hours the gap may be difficult to palpate, and the long flexors to the toes may produce foot movements that simulate true plantar flexion. However, there is still an inability to stand on tiptoe, and squeezing the calf does not cause plantar flexion of the foot (Thompson test).

Treatment
Partial tears are treated with a long leg plaster for 3–4 weeks with the

foot in plantar flexion. Some authorities believe that only a shoe-raise (2·5 cm or so) will suffice for the same time period; but the author favours the former method because it leads to a more rapid resolution of symptoms and signs, especially local swelling.

Complete tears can be treated *conservatively* or by *surgery*.

CONSERVATIVE TREATMENT
This method relies on the close approximation of the torn tendon ends when the foot is in the plantar flexed position. The limb is immobilized in plaster for 6–8 weeks (Lea and Smith, 1972).

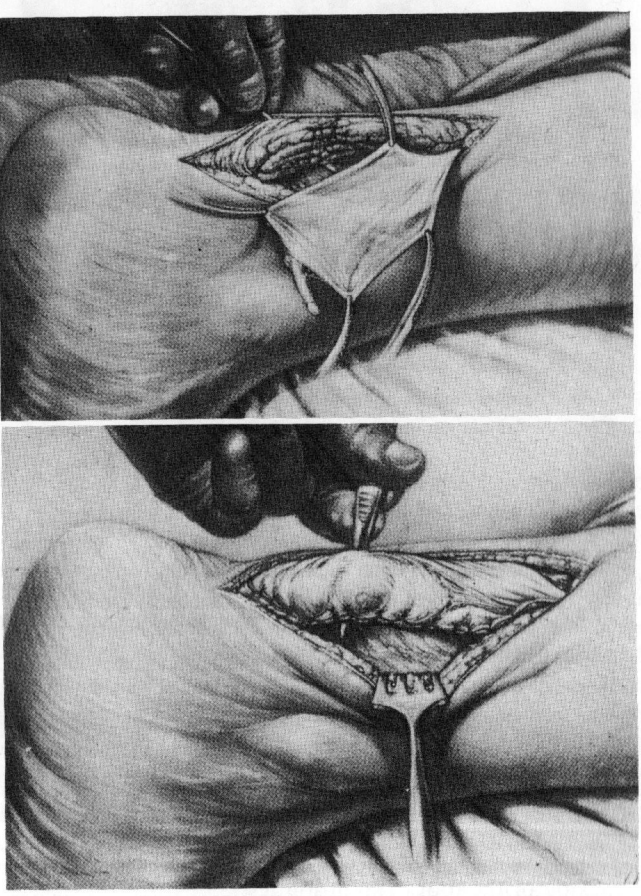

Fig. 13. The tear in the Achilles tendon has been sutured after the ends have been trimmed and the defect is being covered with the fanned-out plantaris tendon (Lynn, 1966).

SURGERY

This is performed as soon after injury as possible. The frayed tendon edges are excised and the tendon repaired with dexon with a wire-pull-out suture to absorb most of the stress. Dexon, wire, fascial strips, plantaris tendon (*Fig.* 13), pieces of the proximal part of the Achilles tendon (Lindholm, 1959) and black silk sutures have been advocated (Crenshaw, 1971). A plaster is applied postoperatively with the foot in equinus and at 3 weeks it is changed and the pull-out wire removed. A new plaster is applied to the lower limb with the foot placed at a right angle; immobilization is continued for a further 3 weeks. Then mobilization exercises are commenced; however, the initial swelling around the Achilles tendon may require ice-facilitation exercises and warm contrast bathing. Sport can usually begin when ankle movements are full and powerful, commonly at 6–9 months from the original injury.

Occasionally a partial tear is encountered at surgery and the gap can be sutured with dexon or similar material. Williams (1976) believes that when a repair is carried out the paratenon should be left unless diseased.

An objective assessment of conservative and surgical treatment of Achilles tendon rupture has been reported by Inglis et al. (1975). They compared 48 cases treated surgically with 28 cases treated non-surgically. They found that plantar flexion was almost one-third weaker in the conservative group and although the surgery-treated patients had no recurrence, 7 patients in the non-surgical group had re-rupture. There was an incidence of 5 per cent wound infection after surgery. Thus there seems little doubt that formal repair of a torn Achilles tendon is the treatment of choice.

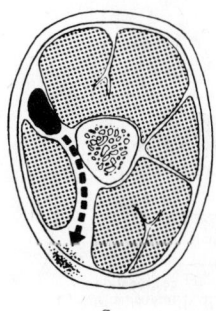   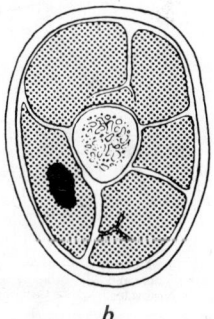

a   *b*

Fig. 14. *a*, Intermuscular haematoma, the blood has tracked down intermuscular fascial planes and appears as bruising often at a site distant from the original injury. *b*, Intramuscular haematoma absorbs more slowly, can usually be palpated but very rarely aspirated.

MUSCLE INJURIES

Injuries to the muscles are caused by direct blows (such as a kick to the thigh, 'Charley-horse injury') or indirect forces (such as a pulled groin).

A muscle haematoma may be intermuscular, intramuscular or mixed (*Fig.* 14). The complications are outlined in *Figs.* 15 and 16.

Diagnosis
Pain, tenderness and spasm occur in the affected muscle. A lump may be palpable.

Treatment
The ICE rule is applied for 20–40 minutes; the limb is rested in a crêpe-and-wool support or a plaster back-slab and inspected at 48 hours. Usually intermuscular injuries show signs of resolution, i.e. less swelling and tenderness, and bruising which may have tracked down fascial planes to appear at some distance from the original injury.

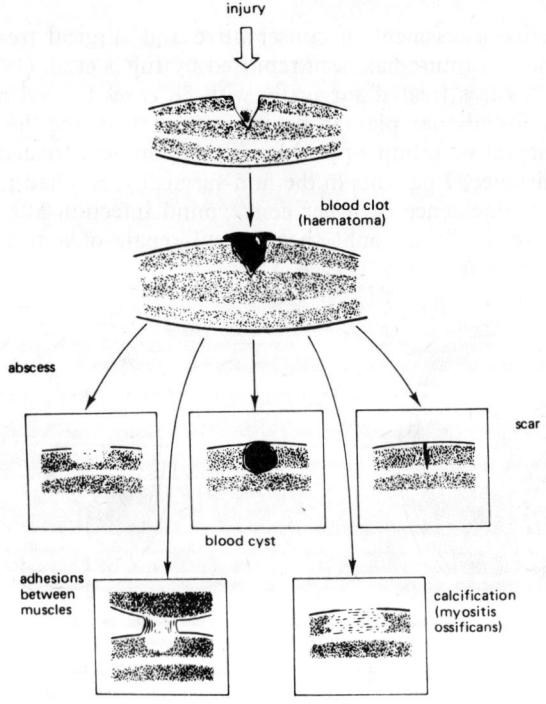

Fig. 15. Stages following a muscle injury.

Intramuscular injuries usually take two or three times longer to resolve; incision may help speed up resolution but is rarely undertaken unless a very large haematoma is found (Tucker and Armstrong, 1964). Aspiration is rarely successful. The limb is immobilized until signs and symptoms have abated, then gentle mobilization begins. The sequence of events is static exercises, gentle passive exercises graduating to active exercises with support, then against gravity and finally against the resistance of weights. These exercises may be used for 7–21 days depending on the nature and severity of the injury. Finally, the player begins to jog, straight track-running, turning, and finally running at speed on the flat, up steps and in the sand-pit. During the earlier phase of rehabilitation the injured area should be assessed every 24 hours, any pain or swelling after exercise should mean rest for 1–2 days and then a recommencement in the grade of activity below the one which reproduced the pain or swelling.

The *recovery* of muscle injury has not taken place until *full power, full extensibility* and *a full range of joint movements and skill patterns* have returned. The ability of a muscle group to stretch to its fullest is vital for maximum power, e.g. the sprinter's crouch which stretches all key muscle groups and produces the powerful contraction necessary for a sudden burst. Without full extensibility athletic performance falls and pulled muscles result.

HERNIA OF MUSCLE
This may occur through a fascial sheath usually in the thigh or anterior tibial region. Surgical excision and repair are only rarely required.

MYOSITIS OSSIFICANS
This condition occurs following a musculoskeletal injury, being common in the thigh, elbow, shoulder and ankle. Pathologically, it consists of ossification in a haematoma when there has been periosteal avulsion. It is believed that the periosteal cells proliferate within the blood clot and ossify it. During the acute stage the muscle may be warm and tender. Any manipulative therapy, such as deep friction massage, only adds to the problem.

Serial radiographs will show the new bone formation at 4–6 weeks as a faint cloud of ossification. This tissue gradually becomes denser until it finally assumes the radiological appearance of mature bone (*Fig.* 16) by 3–6 months.

Treatment
During the acute phase the injured area is treated by rest, using a plaster-of-Paris for 2–4 weeks, if necessary; no heat or manipulations are allowed. Remobilization should only commence after pain and

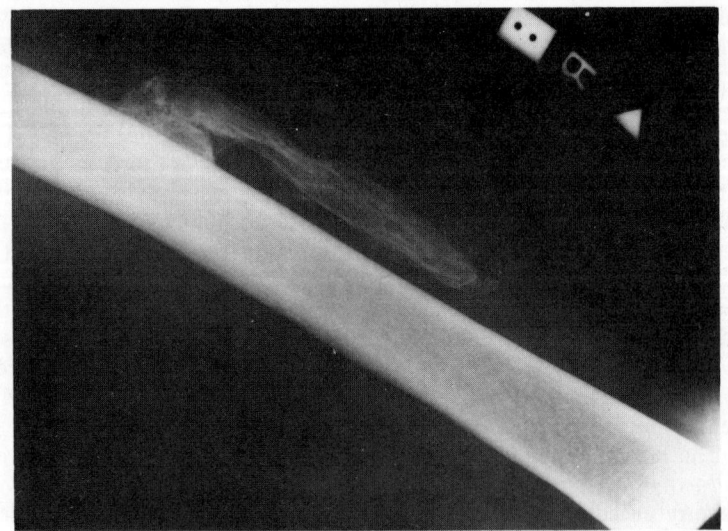

a

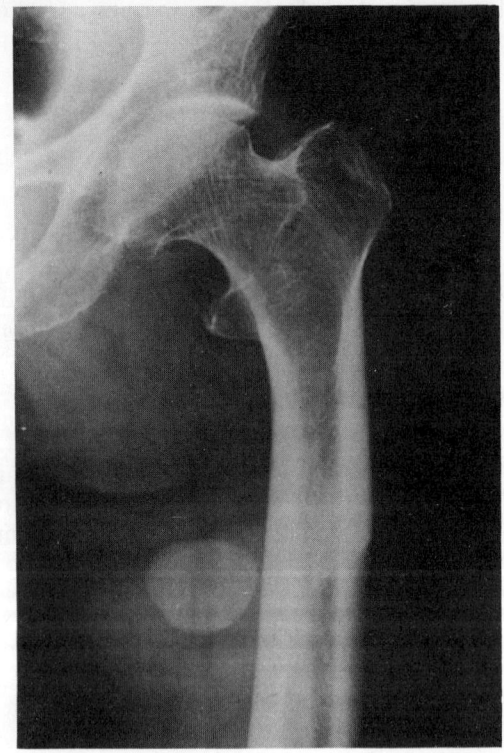

b

tenderness have subsided, and extreme care taken not to provoke further bleeding or swelling. The maturity of the new bone can be assessed by serial radiographs, or a bone scan using a radioactive isotope. When the bone is mature and causing symptoms by pressure, nerve entrapment or friction, it can be excised. In many cases no surgical treatment is needed.

Fig. 16. *a*, Myositis ossificans in the anterior aspect of the thigh—the common site is beneath the vastus intermedius. Early calcification (within weeks of injury) resolves with rest; established lesions may require resection. *b*, An unusual localized (intramuscular) haematoma converted into bone.

Chapter 5

Soft-tissue injuries—chronic

Such injuries may begin with an acute episode or commence insidiously with a gradual deterioration over a period of matches. Many chronic soft-tissue injuries end an athletic career; thus it is essential to prevent them by strict attention to all acute episodes no matter how trivial they appear at the time.

Chronic injuries can be *over-use* injuries (e.g. golfer's elbow), *partial*, but repeated, *tears* (e.g. chronic Achilles' pain) or *incomplete healing* after an *acute episode* (e.g. chronic hamstring injuries). Although each type of injury will be dealt with in turn, the fundamentals of rest, graduated physiotherapy and alteration in style are familiar to all.

CHRONIC SHOULDER PROBLEMS
Tears of Soft Tissues
Tears of the capsular soft tissues and repeated sprains can result in *pericapsulitis* with a limitation of all ranges of shoulder movement; in the extreme a 'frozen shoulder' results. Sometimes an associated hand stiffness is found (*shoulder/hand syndrome*). Cervical spondylosis, brachial neuralgia and tennis elbow may also be present.

TREATMENT
Anti-inflammatory tablets are given for 4 weeks, and a course of 3 or 4 local steroid injections can be used at weekly intervals. Mobilization exercises with short-wave diathermy and ice-facilitation can be very beneficial, but pericapsulitis may persist for 6–9 months, especially after a shoulder dislocation or fracture in the elderly athlete.

Subacromial Bursitis
Lesions of the supraspinatus (Chapter 10) with local calcification can be associated with subacromial bursitis. If a calcified mass is present

on radiography simple surgical removal of this 'toothpaste' material is very effective and can be carried out through a deltoid splitting incision, even under local anaesthetic. Otherwise local steroid injections are used.

Tendinitis of the shoulder is a chronic inflammation of the rotator cuff, most commonly involving the supraspinatus tendon. The action of the shoulder during abduction causes an impingement of the tendons and overlying bursa against the acromion. For this reason partial acromionectomy has been advocated (Leach et al., 1979). This operation involves removal of approximately half of the anterior portion of the acromion. However, since excision of part of the acromion can weaken the deltoid muscle, incision of the coraco-acromial ligament has been described (Jackson, 1976).

CHRONIC ELBOW PROBLEMS
Tennis Elbow
Many conditions produce pain over the lateral aspect of the elbow including cervical spondylosis and radiohumeral osteoarthrosis; however, a true tennis elbow is characterized by pain and tenderness over the common extensor origins on the lateral epicondyle. Pain may also radiate along the course of the extensors in the forearm. The pathology includes subperiosteal haematoma, strain of the extensor origin, calcification and strain of the lateral ligament of the elbow; entrapment of a branch of the radial nerve has been described (Roles and Maudsley, 1972) (*Fig. 17*).

Faults in style and equipment may be found in racket players and fencers. An incorrect size of grip may be incriminated in badminton, tennis and golf, while in some cases a change from a wood to a steel racket may be the cause. In tennis players sliced strokes, especially the wide, low volley with the backhand, are very painful, and the pain is accentuated by all backhand shots and the high-kicking service.

TREATMENT
Local steroids can be given directly into the tender area, weekly for 3–4 weeks. Short-wave diathermy and deep frictions were popular but ultrasound seems to be more effective in the refractory cases. When the pain is acute, immobilization in a plaster back-slab can be used for 2–3 weeks. Tenotomy of the extensor origins, division of the annular ligament, excision of a synovial fringe and radial nerve decompression are only considered in very painful, disabling cases of tennis elbow. Mill's manipulation can be used: the player's fingers and wrist are fully flexed and the forearm pronated, at the same time the elbow is brought into full extension.

Tennis elbow has been described as a self-curing malady (Tucker and Armstrong, 1964) but severe cases may take several months to

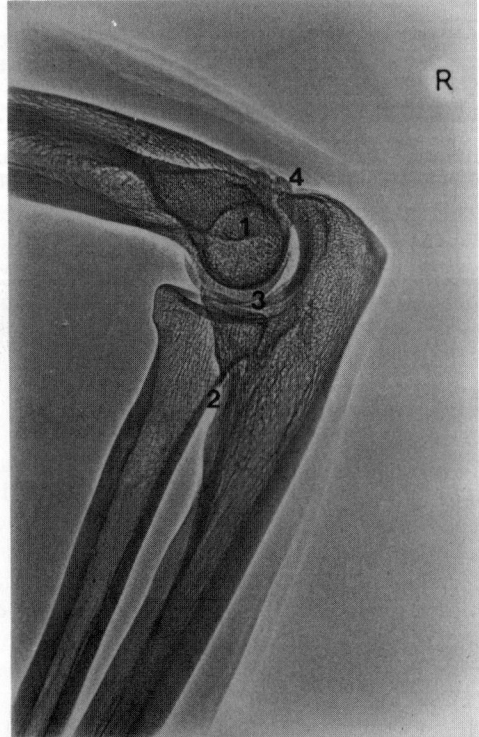

Fig. 17. The painful elbow. 1, Lateral epicondylitis (tennis elbow) (medial epicondylitis equals golfer's elbow); 2, Posterior interosseous nerve entrapment; 3, Lateral ligament strain, or nipping of a synovial fringe or hypertrophic fat pad; 4, Degenerate joint disease, loose bodies, osteochondral fragment, and fracture of an olecranon spur or osteophyte.

abate. A proper warming-up period for 10–20 minutes and a reduction in tennis playing when fatigued will help in the prevention of this refractory condition.

Golfer's Elbow
This condition is the opposite of tennis elbow in that it affects the common flexor origin on the medial side of the elbow. It is due to taking too big a divot in the chip shots and also to a poor grip. The treatment is as for tennis elbow except the manipulation is reversed (the wrist and fingers being extended and the forearm in supination as the elbow is extended).

Baseball Thrower's or Pitcher's Elbow
Some forms of baseball elbow are due to an epicondylitis or epiphysitis in young players ('little league elbow'). However, most elbow injuries

in adult or late adolescent throwers are of the whiplash type and are due to hyperextension at the elbow joint. The result of this hyperextension is that the olecranon impinges in its fossa and a stress fracture may result. Treatment consists of 2-4 weeks' rest and immobilization in plaster, with alteration in style.

Loose bodies and osteophytes, especially on the inner aspect of the trochlea and in the medial ligament, may be found in baseball players. If these outgrowths cause friction on the adjacent soft tissues and ulnar nerve they require enucleation and ligament repair. Baseball pitchers can readily develop swelling of the antecubital muscles because when trying to increase the amount of ball swerve they forcibly supinate the wrist at the termination of the throw. Usually the muscle haemorrhage and oedema settle with rest and immobilization; occasionally myositis ossificans may supervene.

GROIN STRAIN

The commonly affected tendon is the adductor longus at its origin from the pelvis; however, the origins of rectus femoris, sartorius and the iliopsoas may be involved. In all cases the initial injury is the same, namely an unguarded movement at the hip in a fatigued player which tears the muscle at its insertion into bone or tendon (*Fig.* 18).

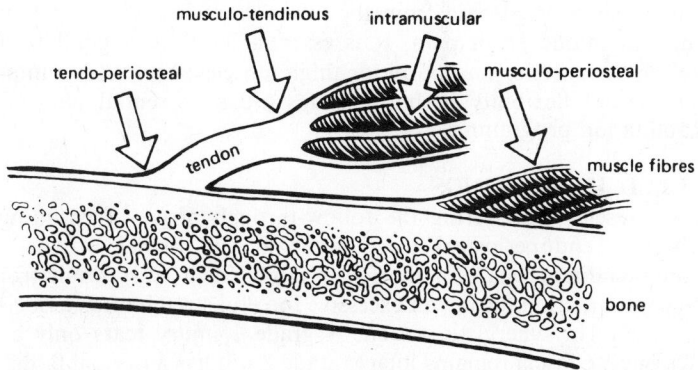

Fig. 18. Indirect muscle injuries occur at the sites indicated; the symptoms of a pulled muscle are often out of all proportion to the clinical signs.

Diagnosis

Bleeding is slight but the pain and loss of function are marked. Local tenderness and muscle spasm will be found and stretching the involved muscle not only reproduces or aggravates the pain but causes it to radiate into the thigh, principally in the distribution of the obturator nerve.

Treatment
There are no short cuts in the treatment of groin strain which can readily become a chronic condition, especially if the players make a hasty return to full training or match play. It is almost impossible to immobilize the hip without a hip spica. Such a course of immobilization would be impractical, however, and the athlete is encouraged to rest as much as possible and to avoid climbing stairs, long walks, etc. Antiinflammatory tablets and short-wave diathermy can be given for pain relief during the first week. Mobilization should follow gradually and if gentle resistance exercises cause discomfort they should be stopped for several days. Ultrasound and resistance exercises are built into the rehabilitation programme which may cover 3–6 weeks. At 2–3 weeks straight-line running and cutting begins; finally running up steps and in the sand-pit are used when discomfort has abated in the groin. Sometimes in refractory cases it is advantageous to stretch the involved muscle. Although local anaesthetic can be used a short-acting intravenous barbiturate is the best way. Surgery is occasionally needed. A tenotomy or Z-plasty lengthening can be performed, and any adhesions divided. However, there is a distinct link between repeat episodes of groin strain and osteitis pubis, probably due to the local inflammatory changes affecting the periosteum. Thus, it is essential to have repeated radiographs of the pelvis in all cases of chronic groin strain. Also referred pain from the lower thoracic and upper lumbar spine can mimic groin pain. It is essential to have a good balance between the anterior and posterior thigh muscles; exercises to improve strength and flexibility in both groups are an essential part of the rehabilitation programme.

PULLED HAMSTRINGS
These muscles tear during the follow-through phase of sprinting or hurdling. Tendoperiosteal tears occur at the ischial origins, and musculotendinous tears in the lower thigh. Such tears result from a violent contraction during an excessive forceful stretch often associated with failure in synergistic action. A grade 1 injury tears only a few fibres but the fascia remains intact; grade 2 still has a normal fascia but a localized haematoma; grade 3 is a tear of many fibres with partial fascial tearing; grade 4 is a complete muscle and fascia tear. Spasm of the hamstrings may accompany low back problems such as spondylolysis or a chronic disc; and may precede or follow meniscal injury or extirpation as the hamstrings attempt to stabilize a malfunctioning knee.

Diagnosis
Pain and tenderness are found; sometimes the pain may radiate along

the sciatic nerve distribution. Stretching the affected muscle causes discomfort.

Treatment
This is adapted from that described in 'groin strain'. Sometimes the lateral popliteal nerve is found to be adherent to the biceps in dense fibrous scarring. Freeing the nerve relieves the acute discomfort.

ANTERIOR THIGH PAIN
Pain in the anterior thigh muscles can be due to partial or complete tears, especially of the rectus femoris, which heal with adhesions to the adjacent muscles and sometimes trap cutaneous branches of the femoral nerve.

Treatment
Local steroids and ultrasound may be effective, with complete rest from sport for 3–6 weeks. Rarely is division of the adhesions required.

CHRONIC KNEE PAIN
Meniscal and ligamentous problems in the knees are described in Chapters 7 and 8. Jumper's knee, chondromalacia patellae and Osgood–Schlatter's disease are discussed in Chapter 6.

BURSAE
A popliteal bursa may indicate osteoarthritic changes in the knee; if troublesome it can be excised but usually attention is directed towards the treatment of the underlying condition. Prepatellar and infrapatellar bursae require aspiration and a pressure dressing—rarely is excision required. Semimembranosus bursa is found in children and usually disappears without treatment after a few months; in adults excision is often required. Many other bursae are found in relationship to the other knee muscles and their treatment is the same as described for semimembranosus bursa.

ILIOTIBIAL BAND FRICTION SYNDROME
The iliotibial band is an important stabilizer of the knee. Friction syndromes occur at the greater trochanter (beneath the tensor fasciae latae) or more commonly at the lateral femoral condyle. It is frequent in long distance runners. The site of the pain is just above the lateral joint line or at the level of the greater trochanter. The true iliotibial band friction syndrome at the knee is aggravated by downhill running.

Treatment
Rest for 2–3 weeks, a period of 'level' running, ultrasound and local

steroids. In chronic cases the tensor fasciae or the posterior portion of the band can be incised.

ANTERIOR AND POSTERIOR COMPARTMENT SYNDROMES

The muscles in both the anterior and posterior compartments of the leg are covered by fascial sheaths (*Fig.* 19). Fractures or soft-tissue injuries can be accompanied by marked swelling within these compartments and infarction; late fibrosis of these muscles may occur. In acute cases decompression is required.

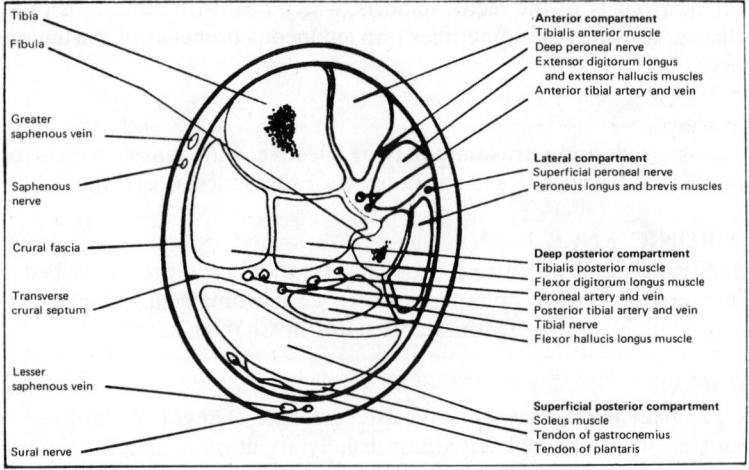

Fig. 19. Cross-sectional anatomy of the leg and its four compartments.

However, most athletic problems in these compartments begin insidiously and are due to the swelling caused by vigorous exercise such as long-distance running on a very hard surface. The tibialis anterior is commonly involved. The affected muscles are very tender. '*Junior leg*' is found in young female gymnasts and is due to soleal hypertrophy and traction on the medial border of the tibia from the attached fascia.

The term '*shin splints*' has been used to describe the overuse pain in the legs due to athletic exertion. There are many causes. *Stress fractures* occur in both the tibia and fibula. The *medial tibial syndrome* is due to muscle hypertrophy or oedema and subsequent ischaemic changes on long distance running. Typically, these pains appear during running, particularly at the toe-off moment and disappear with rest. A localized tender nodular area is found at the medial border of the tibia. However, chronic ischaemic changes may also occur in other fascial compartments of the leg. The *anterior compartment syndrome* has discomfort and tenderness located on the anterolateral side of the leg (Orava and Puranen, 1979). Although asymptomatic at rest, patients experience a painful, tight sensation with weakness on dorsiflexion, and occasional paraesthesiae on the dorsum of the foot, after exercise. Physical examination at rest is often normal but generally muscle tenderness and weakness increases with activity. Common conditions which should be excluded are claudication from peripheral vascular disease, tendinitis and fatigue fractures. Pain which occurs with the first few steps but can be 'run off' is not due to a compartmental syndrome.

Treatment
Rest, elevation, massage and short-wave diathermy appear to be the most effective methods. A gradual build-up in training methods, the provision of well-fitting rubber shoes to absorb the stresses initially and the avoidance of hard surfaces are all used. A radiograph or isotope studies must be taken of the tibia and fibula to exclude a stress fracture (which is treated by rest for 3–6 weeks). The thickened fascia can be divided for decompression in 'junior leg'; the insertion of the fascia on the medial border of the tibia can be released using a fasciotome inserted through a small posterior incision medial to the gastrocnemius/soleus muscles. Once areas of necrosis and fibrosis (especially involving small radicles of the anterior or posterior tibial nerve) have developed the condition is very refractory to treatment.

Periostitis typically occurs on the medial side of the leg and is due to small subperiosteal haemorrhages and swelling. Common in footballers the treatment is by local steroids and a local anaesthetic (usually one or two injections).

CHRONIC ACHILLES TENDON LESIONS
Repeated trauma due to overuse or direct injury will cause areas of focal degeneration within the Achilles tendon, leading to a weakening of its structural strength and ultimate rupture. Ismail et al. (1969) have emphasized the importance of local steroids in weakening collagen, thus leading to eventual rupture. The author does not favour local steroid injections into the Achilles (or other) tendons (*Fig.* 20).

Chronic pain in the region of the Achilles tendon can be due to thickening of the paratenon as well as focal degeneration, and usually both coexist.

Although heat and mobilization exercises, padding of the heel and ultrasound can be used in the early forms of Achilles pain, refractory lesions may require surgery. The tendon is exposed and the paratenon removed over 80 per cent of its circumference. The lesion is identified and the tendon divided in its long axis down and through the focal degeneration. This tissue and the granulation tissue are removed with

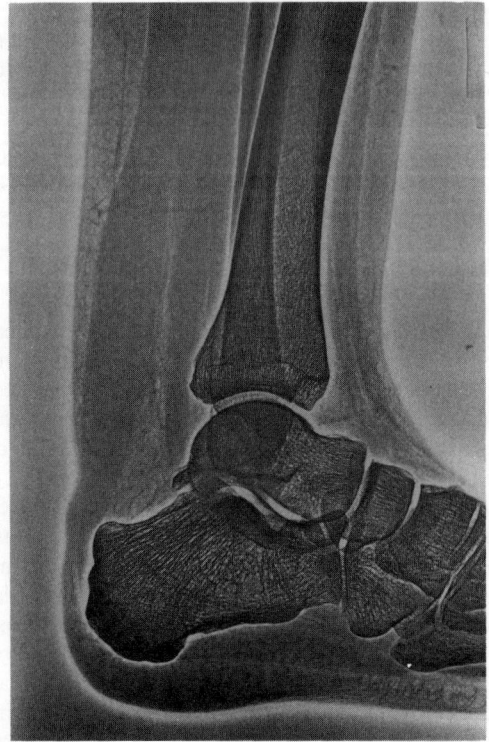

Fig. 20. Gross thickening of the Achilles tendon due to fibrosis around a healed (almost complete) tear in a female badminton player (aged 36 years).

a curette and the wound is closed in layers. The player remains in bed for 4 days but ankle movements are encouraged, particularly dorsiflexion. On the second to fifth postoperative days the player gets up and begins weight-bearing, using a soft slipper. Progress with weight-bearing is as rapid as the patient can tolerate. After about 3 weeks the player can begin normal training.

A common cause of pain at the insertion of the Achilles tendon into the heel is due to a small bursa and either this can be infiltrated with local steroids or an ultrasound used. Sometimes a small spur of bone is found and surgical excision of the spur and bursa is carried out.

The prevention of Achilles lesions requires sorbo-rubber insoles, a slightly raised heel on the sports shoes, a ban on the wearing of very high-heeled shoes during everyday life (thus reducing the contrast between sports shoe heels and normal heels) and the avoidance of training on hard surfaces, including gym floors (*Fig.* 21).

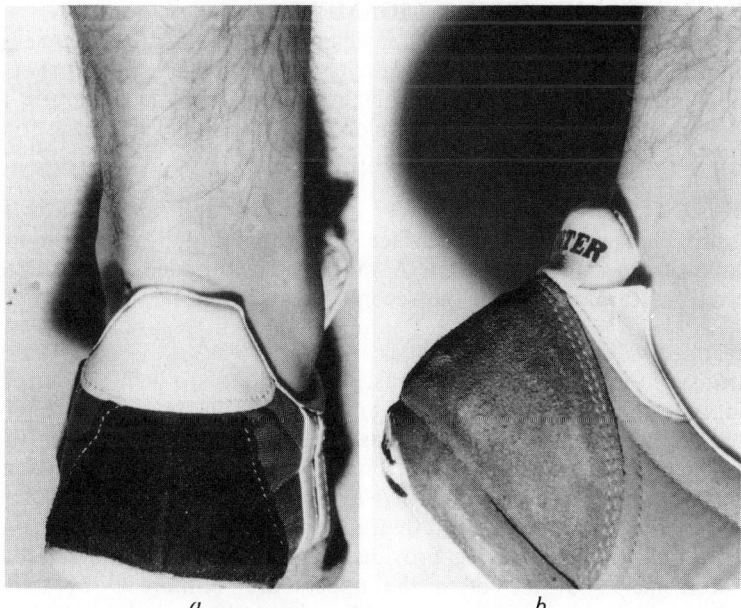

Fig. 21. A common cause of Achilles tendinitis. *a*, Due to the so-called Achilles protector. *b*, The remedy is shown (also note the worn down and level heel which could also predispose to problems).

CHRONIC ANKLE PROBLEMS

Spikes or studs that give excessive grip on the field or track predispose to ankle injuries and chronic sprains. In footballers a traumatic osteitis is found due to repeated dead-ball kicking (Chapter 9).

BRUISED HEEL

This complaint is common amongst hurdlers and long and triple jumpers. Repeated heavy landings on the heels cause rupture of the fibrous septa between the skin and calcaneus so that the protective fatty layer becomes dissipated, and local pain and tenderness are found. The treatment consists of a thick, soft sponge-rubber or plastazote heel pad. However, a moulded heel cup may also be used; this cup is designed to compress the lateral aspects of the heel and prevents displacement of the soft tissue.

PLANTAR FASCIITIS

Local tenderness is found beneath the heel and a calcaneal spur may be seen on radiography. In early cases local steroids, heel padding and ultrasound may be effective, but chronic cases require excision of the spur or incision of the plantar fascia close to the calcaneus.

SPRAIN OF THE SPRING LIGAMENT
Sprains of the plantar calcaneonavicular ligament (spring ligament) may follow unaccustomed running over uneven surfaces in soft shoes. The clinical picture is similar to plantar fasciitis but the tenderness is more anterior and medial. A moulded felt insole and instrinsic foot exercises with ultrasound are required.

CHRONIC FOOT STRAIN
Unsuitable shoes and hard surfaces can cause a dull ache over the whole of the sole of the foot. A radiograph is needed to exclude a march fracture, usually in the second metatarsal neck.

Treatment
Intrinsic foot exercises and contrast foot bathing are helpful. Correct footwear should be worn both in an event and in training but badly sited studs can cause pressure areas and provoke sesamoiditis at the first metatarsal heads. Worn-out boots or shoes which are 'trodden-over' or whose soles have given way are a frequent source of foot trouble. Players should ensure that good footwear is light, supple and well fitting. Extra support is provided by the careful siting of suitable reinforcement but too often the uppers are 'reinforced' by trade flashes which cause rubbing and blistering. Cleats, spikes or studs improve adhesion, but it is useless to have studs that do not go into the ground, leaving the sole of the foot unsupported. Multiple short studs are much more safe and effective on grass than a few long studs. However, a rigid sole under the forefoot and tight uppers will prevent the transference of weight by the ankle from one arch of the foot to the other; thus ankle problems are common especially with the popular polyurethane rigid soles. Nylon is a most unsuitable material as it is unyielding and frequently bends in the wrong place (i.e. half-way along the sole and not under the metatarsophalangeal joints) and it is easily scored by sharp stones, etc. Leather boots and soles give good flexibility and the studs should transmit weight without causing pressure areas. Nylon and rubber studs have metal tips which protrude once the overlying material has worn; thus studs should be checked regularly.

Chapter 6

Injuries to the thigh and knee

This chapter deals principally with bony injuries in these regions.

DISLOCATION OF THE HIP
Posterior dislocation is more common than anterior and the sciatic nerve is liable to damage. Fragments may be detached from the margins of the acetabulum or a fracture may extend into the pelvic bones. Occasionally a central dislocation occurs. Since the hip joint is both strong and stable great force is required to produce such injuries, being common in high-speed vehicular accidents and sometimes with horse-riding accidents. Posterior dislocations usually occur with a force transmitted to the knee with the hip flexed and adducted.

Diagnosis
Great pain, muscle spasm and an inability to move the hip are present while paraesthesia and weakness may be found in the distribution of the sciatic nerve.

Treatment
Reduction requires general anaesthesia and muscle relaxation. The hip is usually easily reduced with flexion and adduction followed by gentle traction. However, surgery may be needed to remove loose bodies and to reconstruct the acetabular margins.
    Fractures of the femoral head or upper femoral shaft may complicate hip dislocations. Avascular necrosis of the femoral head occurs in 20 per cent of cases.

FRACTURES OF THE FEMUR
Femoral Neck
Stress fractures of the femoral neck occur in athletes and running is forbidden for 4–6 months, because there is a risk of displacement.

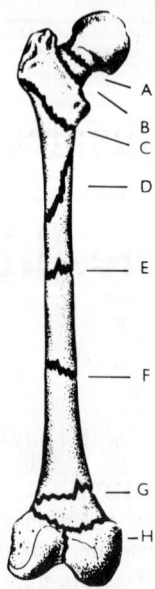

Fig. 22. Fractures of the femur commonly found in athletes. A, Transcervical; B, Basal cervical; C, Trochanteric; D, Spiral shaft; E, Transverse; F, Oblique; G, Supracondylar; H, Condylar T-shaped.

Femoral Shaft Fractures

A spiral fracture is caused by a fall in which the foot is anchored, while direct trauma causes a transverse fracture (*Fig.* 22).

DIAGNOSIS

Severe pain, swelling of the thigh and a shocked state make the diagnosis obvious. At least 1 litre of blood may be lost into the thigh.

TREATMENT

Immediate splinting of the limb is performed and the player is removed on a stretcher. After a blood transfusion has been set up the fracture is reduced under general anaesthesia. Conservative treatment is the use of a Thomas splint for 12 weeks. With fractures of the lower half of the femur a weight-relieving calliper or a Sarmiento plaster can be used after 6-8 weeks to mobilize the player if consolidation is taking place. While on traction patellar and knee movements are encouraged.

Surgery

This method is very effective in athletes and leads to early mobilization of the knee with only 3 weeks of bed rest in most cases. Fractures of the upper third and transverse fractures in the mid-shaft are suitable for internal fixation with a Küntscher nail; lower fractures may be treated with a compression plate. Internal reduction is also required when closed reduction has failed due to soft-tissue interposition or when another fracture (usually the tibia) occurs in the same limb. Weight-bearing can begin at 4–6 months depending on the nature of the fracture and the speed of healing; it is wise to have a further 1–3 months of partial weight-bearing with crutches and later a stick before returning to full activity. These measures prevent refracture or anterior bowing of the femur. Sport can begin again between 12 and 18 months; if intramedullary fixation has been performed the nail is removed at 12–18 months before training is fully completed.

SUPRACONDYLAR AND CONDYLAR FRACTURES
The supracondylar fracture (*Fig.* 22) is usually caused by a direct blow; the lower fragment may be tilted backwards by the gastrocnemius. Femoral condylar fractures (*Fig.* 22) may be caused by direct trauma or a fall from a height which drives the tibia into the intercondylar fossa. In an adolescent the lower femoral epiphysis may be displaced in rugby or by a heavy tackle in American football—condylar fractures are fairly common in this sport and the knee ligaments are also injured.

Diagnosis
The knee is swollen and deformed and all movements are painful. The pulses below the knee should be checked to make sure that the popliteal vessels are not obstructed.

Treatment
Epiphysial injuries are treated conservatively with a Thomas splint and traction for 6–12 weeks unless undisplaced, when a long-leg plaster is used for 6 weeks. In adults internal fixation is used if closed reduction is poor or if early knee mobilization is desired—a right-angled blade-plate or lag-screws being used in condylar fractures. In all cases the haemarthrosis must be aspirated. Knee stiffness is a problem following all femoral shaft fractures and can end an athletic career. Thus quadriceps exercises are an integral part of the early treatment; knee flexion being encouraged and facilitated by using a knee-piece attachment to the splint or a divided mattress. Tethering of the quadriceps to the fracture site may limit knee flexion and necessitate a quadricepsplasty or an elongation of the extensor mechanism.

FRACTURED PATELLA
The patella is commonly fractured by a direct blow which knocks it against the femur (*Fig.* 23) although the expansion on each side usually remains intact. However, a sudden contraction of the quadriceps may cause a transverse avulsion fracture and this expansion is torn.

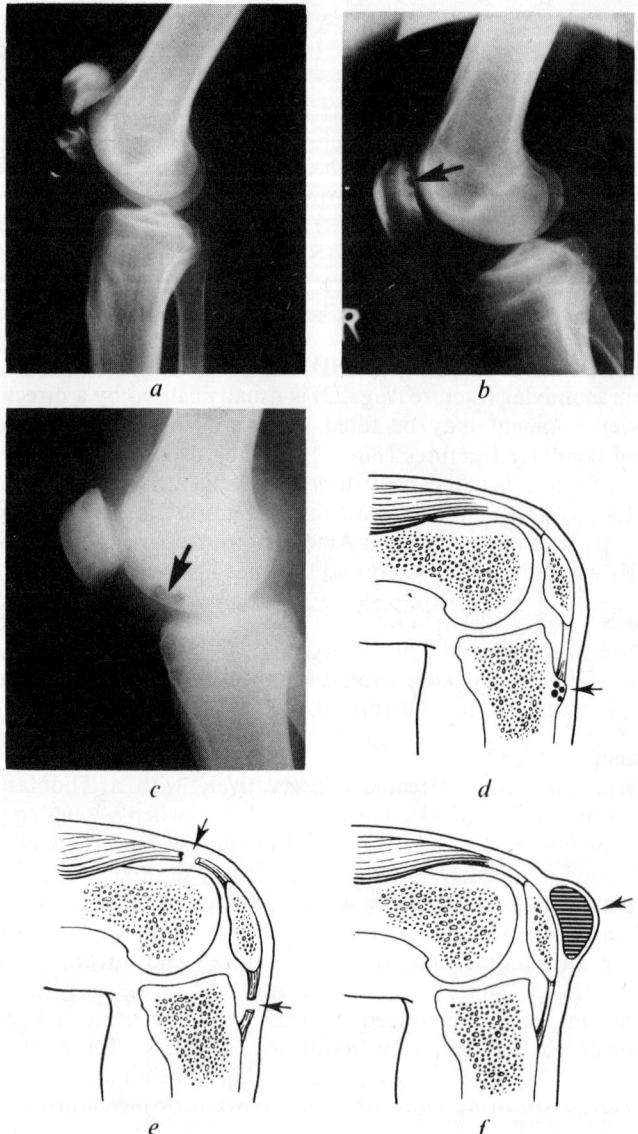

Fig. 23. Causes of knee pain in athletes. *a*, Transverse fracture of the patella (direct injury). *b*, Osteoarthritic changes in the patellar cartilage. *c*, Osteochondritis dissecans in an adolescent athlete. *d*, Osgood–Schlatter's disease of the tibial tubercle in an adolescent. *e*, Tears in the quadriceps expansion and patellar tendon (indirect injury). *f*, Prepatellar swelling. May be due to bursitis or, in acute cases, a small bleed into the bursa (this can be associated with a crack fracture of the patella).

Diagnosis
The knee is swollen and the patellar tendon has a palpable gap.

Treatment
Undisplaced fractures are treated conservatively with a plaster cylinder for 3–4 weeks. However, displaced fragments require reduction and fixation with wires or screws; reduction must be accurate or the femoral condyles will be scored. Although small pieces can be excised, a patellectomy is carried out if a comminuted fracture is found. When the extensor expansion is torn it must be repaired or else an extension lag of 10–20° will occur. Patellectomy results in a 25–45 per cent loss of knee efficiency and in footballers there is a marked loss of power in dead-ball kicking, but in some sports, e.g. cricket and golf, activity can be maintained to a good standard.

DISLOCATION OF THE PATELLA
When the knee is extended and the quadriceps is relaxed the patella may be pushed laterally by a blow and dislocate.

Diagnosis
The deformity of the patella is obvious.

Treatment
An initial dislocation is treated by reduction; anaesthesia is not always needed. Quadriceps exercises are begun at once and a plaster cylinder is used for 2–3 weeks. Sport can begin at 4 weeks. In recurrent cases, especially in adolescent girls, a tibial transfer operation or reefing of the quadriceps expansion medially (and a relieving incision laterally) may be performed.

CHONDROMALACIA PATELLAE
Common in adolescent girls, but may be found in cyclists and occasionally in sports such as hockey when a blow to the knee has been an aggravating factor. The articular cartilage loses its normal smooth glistening appearance; in one or more areas it becomes oedematous, dull and soft, so that at operation it is easily indented. Fine irregular fissures or a small erupting area (like a blister) are found at surgery, and not uncommonly a 'kissing' lesion is found on the femoral condyle.

Diagnosis
The patient complains of knee pain, especially on sitting or climbing and the knee may give way. Grating and tenderness are found when the patella is pressed against the femoral condyles. Valgus knees, external tibial torsion and 'squinting' patellae are associated conditions (*Fig.* 24).

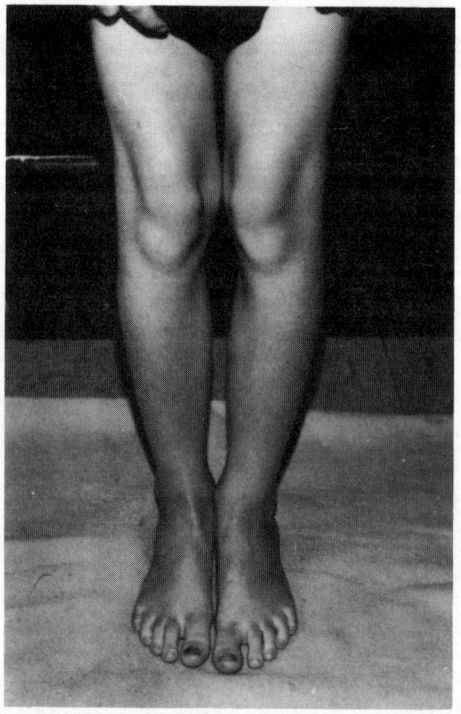

Fig. 24. 'Kissing' or 'squinting' patellae: associated with chondromalacia patellae, tibial torsion and pronated feet.

Treatment
Sport is stopped for 1–3 months and vigorous quadriceps exercises performed. Analgesics are given to relieve pain. A lateral retinacular release is often effective, but if symptoms are severe an arthrotomy is carried out. Excision of the softened area can be performed and with patellar realignment gave 79 per cent good results in 87 knees (Insall et al., 1976). Severe cases warrant patellectomy. After retinacular release sport can begin at 8–12 weeks.

MEDIAL SYNOVIAL PLICA
The medial synovial plica is a fold of synovium that extends from the superomedial aspect of the patella distally to insert into the infrapatellar fat pad. When thickened it forms a restrictive band across the medial condyle during knee flexion and can alter patellar mechanics, giving pain on climbing stairs as well as other symptoms of chondromalacia patellae. Conservative measures of rest, anti-inflammatory agents and isometric exercises usually suffice but in refractory cases the plica must be excised either by arthroscopic or arthrotomy procedures.

BIPARTITE PATELLA
This congenital condition is occasionally a cause of knee pain and secondary chondromalacia, particularly if a small piece is misaligned. Sometimes excision of the piece is justified. A bipartite patella should be differentiated from a fracture.

OSGOOD-SCHLATTER'S DISEASE
The epiphysis of the anterior tibial tubercle (*Fig.* 23) becomes infarcted due to excessive pull from the patellar tendon. It is common in boys of 10–16 years and usually only persists for a few months, for once the epiphysis fuses the condition abates. One month in a plaster cylinder or 1–3 months off games usually suffices. Although local steroid injections can be effective, rarely is shaving of the tibial tubercle required unless there is excessive local tenderness or a hypertrophic mass of bone.

SINDING-LARSEN-JOHANNSON DISEASE
This is a rare osteochondritis of the lower pole of the patella and is treated in the same way as Osgood–Schlatter's disease, although excision of the lower pole of the patella is seldom justified.

PELLEGRINI-STIEDA'S DISEASE
This consists of heterotopic calcification in the upper fibres of the medial collateral ligament; local tenderness and pain on springing the knee may be found. Local steroid injections offer relief; occasionally the calcified lump requires excision. This condition may be due to faulty healing following partial avulsion of the upper attachment of the medial collateral ligament.

JUMPER'S KNEE
This is an amalgamation of several of the conditions described. The athlete is almost always involved in some type of repetitive activity such as jumping, climbing, kicking or running. The common sports with this complication are basketball, volleyball, high jumping, long and triple jumping, football, figure skating, tennis, climbing and long-distance running.

Diagnosis
There is often a pain of insidious onset over the infrapatellar or suprapatellar regions and the pain disappears with rest. A sensation of weakness, giving way and fullness around the knee are described (Blazina, 1973).

When the symptoms are marked and the athlete persists with sports an acute episode, namely a 'giving way' of the knee, is experienced;

occasionally there may be a complete rupture of the tendinous attachment to the involved pole.
The poles of the patella or the patellar tendon may be tender. Effusion is rare but sometimes there may be a snapping sensation of the patella on full knee flexion. The athlete is usually tall and there may be abnormalities of the extensor mechanism such as patellar hypermobility and subluxation, patella alta, Osgood–Schlatter's disease, chondromalacia patellae, genu recurvatum, genu valgum and external tibial torsion. Radiography may be normal but occasionally shows rarefaction at the involved pole.

Treatment
Rest for 2–4 weeks, anti-inflammatory agents and a long elastic knee support can be given, but in refractory cases plaster immobilization for 3–4 weeks is used. Surgery may be required and a variety of procedures are carried out. These include drilling of the involved pole, resection of the involved pole, excision of any degenerate tendon, reattachment of the patellar tendon and retinacular reinforcement (Blazina, 1973). Sport may be resumed after 6 months.

OSTEOCHONDRITIS DISSECANS
Only convex surfaces are affected and trauma is the most likely cause of this osteochondral or stress fracture.

Diagnosis
The patient, aged between 15 and 20 years, presents with vague knee pains or swelling and a tender medial condyle (rarely lateral). Later the knee may give way or lock. A radiograph shows the ovoid segment on the medial condyle close to the anterior tibial spine, while sometimes a small crater and loose body may be seen.

Treatment
In the earliest stages the knee can be treated conservatively but usually surgery is needed. The fragment (*Fig.* 23c) can be fixed with small pins or, more commonly, excised. (The capitellum, talus, femoral head and first metatarsal head may also be sites of this disorder.)

Chapter 7

Meniscal damage in the knee

Injuries to the menisci of the knees are a common problem in sportsmen. With the advent of better diagnostic aids such as arthrography and arthroscopy much information has been gathered about the specific function of the menisci as well as the pathological processes involved.

FUNCTIONS
The menisci act as shock absorbers, allow the femur to glide as well as rotate relative to the tibia and are stabilizers of the knee. One of the chief functions that has not been appreciated is the role the menisci play in the control of rotatory instability and shear.

INJURY TO THE MENISCI
1. A horizontal cleavage lesion occurs with degenerative changes in the menisci and knee; it may be associated with minor repetitive trauma such as repeated squatting or climbing.
2. The vertical, oblique or longitudinal tear is caused by a force grinding the meniscus between the femur and tibia; characteristically this occurs when: (*i*) weight is being taken, (*ii*) the knee is flexed, and (*iii*) there is a twisting strain. This type of lesion is common in sportsmen and sportswomen.
3. Fraying or other signs of attrition may be found in association with ligamentous laxity, especially the medial collateral and anterior cruciate ligaments. Ultimately frank degenerative changes or tearing result.

Diagnosis
A torn meniscus can cause little or no symptoms in the earliest stages

or conversely the tear becomes apparent in an acute episode. Commonly pain is experienced localized to the joint line; generally the discomfort localizes to the affected side but in some instances the discomfort may be deep seated and ill-defined. There may be loss of movement of a few degrees—usually at the extremes of flexion and extension—while swelling and wasting of the vastus medialis may be seen. An important sign is tenderness over the affected joint line. Sometimes a cyst may be felt. Such symptoms and signs are common with degenerative, frayed or slightly torn menisci. However, when a large tear is produced the torn piece may become displaced and cause locking; a locked knee will usually flex but not extend, occasionally muscle spasm prevents both movements. With extension the tibial tubercle should move laterally relative to the patella; this does not occur if the knee is locked (Helfet's sign). The patient may also note a clicking or clunking on moving the affected knee.

Between attacks the tenderness and pain may disappear and the player often returns to sport. This is common after posterior horn tears which rarely cause locking and present with a dull ache in the posterior part of the joint.

In McMurray's test for a medial meniscus damage the foot is externally rotated and the flexed knee straightened, and as the bony surfaces pass over the torn cartilage a click may be heard or a jump felt by the fingers resting on the joint line. With lateral meniscus tears the leg is gently extended from full flexion with internal rotation of the foot. Apley's grinding test with the patient face down and the knee flexed at a right angle depends on the fact that when the tibia is pushed on to the femoral condyles the ligaments are relaxed and grinding of the torn meniscus causes pain; distraction releases the meniscus but stretches the ligaments and causes pain if these are injured.

It is worth noting that both of these tests can be negative in the presence of meniscal lesions. The most important way to reach a diagnosis is from the history. Usually the player is darting forwards with his weight on a flexed knee, at this time due to a body check or in trying to avoid an opponent, the knee is rotated and the meniscus is thus trapped between the femoral condyles and tibial plateau. Under normal circumstances the meniscus would rapidly move away from the advancing femur, but if the retaining structures are weakened or the attachments are lax the meniscus is trapped and torn. On other occasions the player is banged or tackled heavily from the side and along with a severe ligament strain or tear the cartilage is split. Strangely enough this is one of the few soccer injuries which can occur in the dressing room, the knee suddenly locking as the player straightens from tying his boots.

AIDS TO DIAGNOSIS
A plain radiograph should be taken to exclude loose bodies and fractures.

Arthrography is extremely useful, and a negative arthrogram frequently means that the symptoms are due to some other condition, especially if pseudo-locking has been a feature. Arthrograms are 95 per cent effective in medial meniscus lesions and 85 per cent in lateral meniscus lesions (Nicholas, 1973a). The presence of a discoid meniscus may be confirmed by arthrography, and this test will outline cruciate lesions, popliteal cysts, capsular laxity and tears.

Arthroscopy may show meniscal tears most effectively as well as other intra-articular pathology. It is usually reserved for knees which do not have a clear history of a meniscal injury, when the arthrogram is of doubtful value or, being negative, conflicts with the clinical impression, when other pathology could be causing the symptomatology rather than the meniscus and in persisting knee problems after surgery, including meniscectomy. It is, however, a skilled procedure and requires a small incision.

THE LOCKED KNEE
A radiograph is taken to exclude loose bodies, osteochondritis dissecans, and a fractured tibial spine. A recurrent dislocation of the patella must be excluded.

The knee is manipulated, if necessary, under general anaesthesia. The joint is fully rotated in varying degrees of flexion until full extension is obtained. Sometimes spurious unlocking is achieved because the torn fragment slips into the intercondylar fossa. A plaster backslab or cylinder is worn in full extension for 2–3 weeks, then the player begins training again.

In the author's experience surgery is rarely required for the first acute episode; meniscectomy is required if there is incomplete knee mobility. This sometimes happens when the player presents days or even weeks after the acute episode.

Pseudo-locking
This may be due to chondromalacia patellae, injuries of the infrapatellar fat pad and ligamentous injuries, including coronary ligament sprains, also to an exostosis of the femur (*Fig.* 25).

HORIZONTAL OR DEGENERATIVE LESION
The horizontal cleavage lesion in a degenerative meniscus was first fully described by Smillie (1973). In his department these tears accounted for almost 50 per cent of the menisci removed. Horizontal

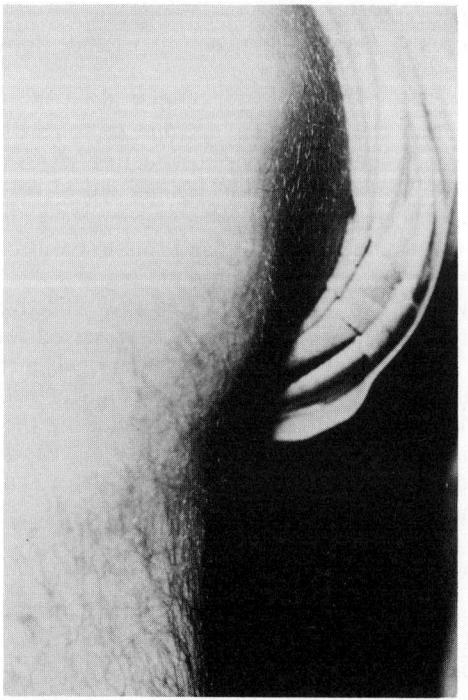

Fig. 25. An exostosis of the femur causing 'pseudo-locking' by impingement with the medial hamstring tendons.

lesions are common in the older sportsmen whose knees show evidence of osteoarthrosis. Noble and Hamblen (1975) found that these lesions were twice as common in the medial as in the lateral meniscus, whereas in their series osteoarthrosis was more common in the lateral compartment. They believed that the two conditions may often coexist rather than be causally related. Horizontal lesions were commoner in males and in large menisci, and 18 per cent showed calcification in the above series.

Treatment
If the symptoms can be traced to the degenerative meniscus (usually pain and tenderness localized to the joint line with a feeling of instability on climbing or squatting) the offending meniscus can be removed.

TORN MEDIAL MENISCUS
Fig. 26 depicts the varieties of tears in the meniscus.
Fig. 27 shows the lesion as seen at arthrography and arthroscopy.

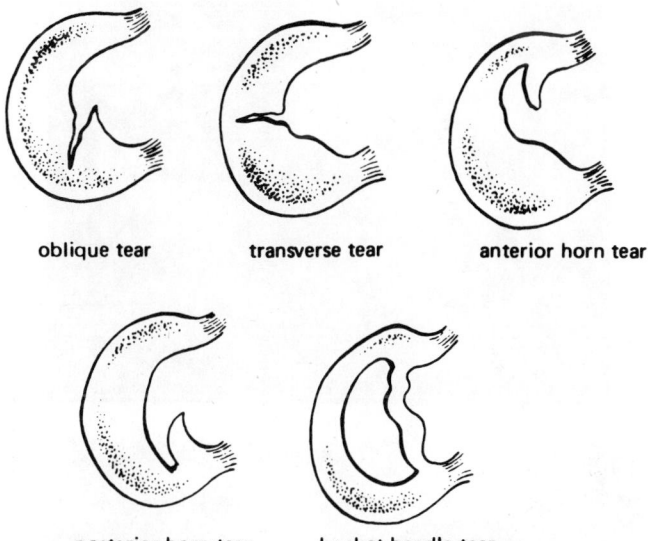

Fig. 26. Meniscal injuries.

Treatment

The initial acute episode can be treated conservatively (*see above*, Locked Knee) but repeated episodes require excision of the meniscus. However, medial meniscectomy should not be regarded as an innocent procedure. When there is anterior cruciate laxity the meniscus may actually be providing some stability. Degenerative changes in the knee may be produced by meniscectomy especially if a relatively normal meniscus is removed. Meniscectomy is often characterized by the failure to recover full flexion; while hyperalgesia or anaesthesia of the infrapatellar nerve may be troublesome.

A painful, swollen knee, with repeated episodes of locking and tenderness over the femoral condyles indicative of attrition from the torn meniscus, warrants meniscectomy. Small tears found in the anterior and posterior horn at arthrography do not warrant this operation.

A small anteromedial incision is used. The most difficult problem is to remove a torn posterior horn, especially where a bucket-handle tear extends to the periphery, and a further posterior incision may have to be made. When a flap of meniscus extends into the intercondylar area and the remaining rim appears to be firmly attached to the capsule then the offending piece of meniscus is excised and the peripheral part left.

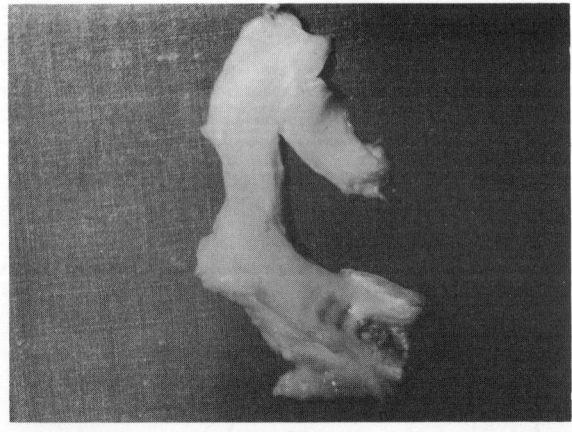

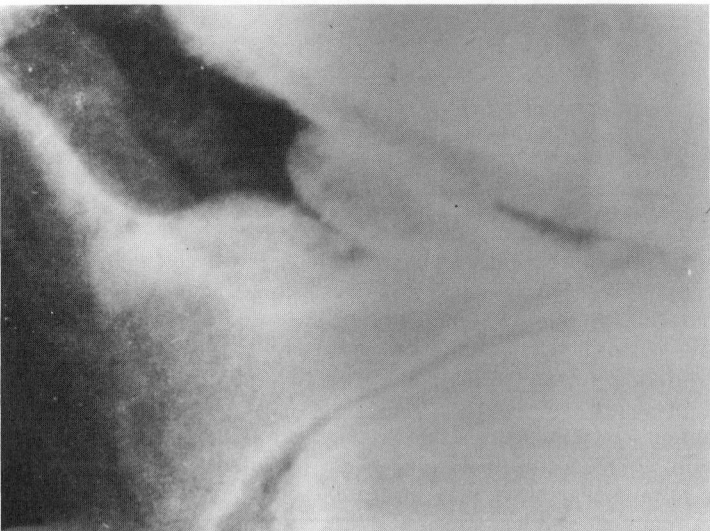

Fig. 27. *a*, An oblique tear of the medial meniscus. *b*, At arthrography. *c*, *d*, At arthroscopy.

TORN LATERAL MENISCUS

The lateral meniscus is less liable to tear because its attachments permit more mobility; injury is followed by pain and instability but locking is uncommon.

More frequently the lateral meniscus develops a cyst and the characteristic lump is easily seen and felt on the outer aspect of the knee.

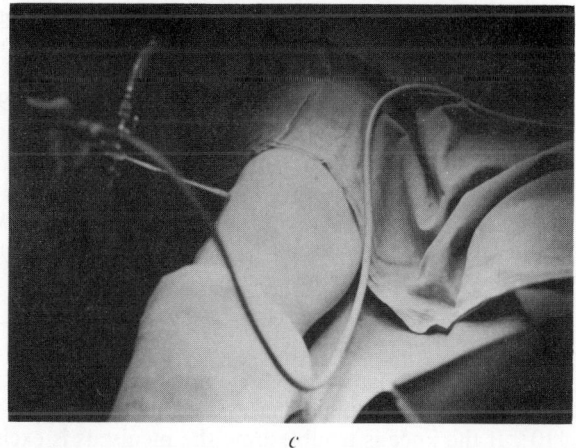

c

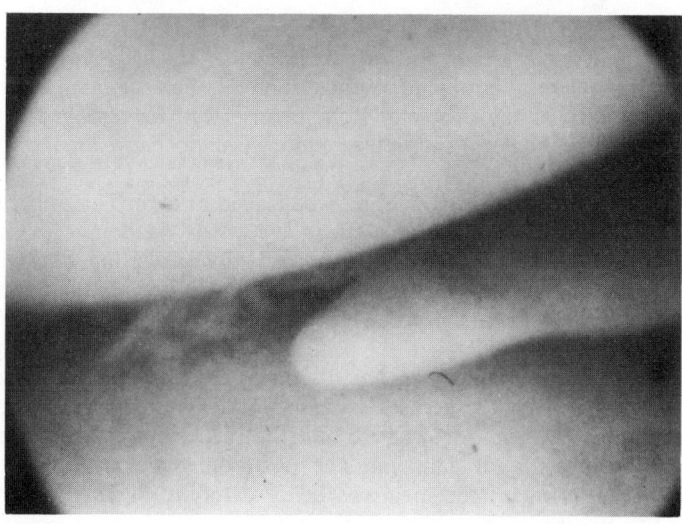

d

Treatment
It is more difficult to expose the lateral meniscus because of its anterior cruciate fixation, overlying fat pad and circular structure. An anterolateral incision or the Bruser incision can be used and sometimes the lateral meniscus is better removed with the knee in extension or in 10° of flexion in contradistinction to the 135° of flexion used on the

medial side. Care must be taken not to cut the lateral geniculate artery which is quite variable in size and location or a severe haemarthrosis or false aneurysm may occur.

When dealing with a cystic meniscus Flynn and Kelly (1976) have described the method of removing only the cystic area and leaving the lateral meniscus behind if it is not torn. The rationale for local excision was based on the similarity between the cyst and a ganglion and also on the desirability of preserving the meniscus. However, when there is doubt about the meniscus a formal arthrotomy has to be carried out with excision of the meniscus.

DISCOID LATERAL MENISCUS
Usually found in young patients who complain that the knee gives way or clunks loudly; this sound may be elicited by flexing the knee to about 110°. If the knee is troublesome the meniscus is excised.

SPECIAL PROBLEMS AND ASSOCIATED LESIONS
Bilateral tears may occur and often the medial meniscus lesion overshadows the lateral problem. Arthrography is helpful in delineating the bilaterality of the problem. Both menisci can be removed at the same time, the bilateral incisions do not seem to carry an increased morbidity.

The anterior cruciate ligament may be frayed or torn. This is because the cruciate ligaments only act effectively when the femur (with its axis of rotation) is allowed to move freely forwards and backwards on the tibia. A torn meniscus blocks this to-and-fro mobility putting stress on these ligaments, especially the anterior, which ultimately tear. Some sports injuries damage the anterior cruciate directly or as part of the triad of medial ligament, medial meniscus and anterior cruciate (*see* Chapter 8). In these cases Nicholas (1973a) advises removal of the stump of the anterior cruciate and the torn meniscus; he stresses the importance of not damaging the posteromedial capsule and the medial compartment, the meniscus being carefully dissected out just lateral to its fibrous capsular attachment.

Degenerative changes may occur in the knee, with or without meniscal problems, and usually the medial femoral condyle or the patellar cartilage is affected. If a popliteal cyst develops, attention should be directed towards the underlying knee problem; simple excision of the cyst is usually unfruitful if effusions recur due to osteoarthritic changes. An intra-articular ganglion or nipping of the fat pad is sometimes found (Muckle, 1972b). A synovial biopsy can be performed if the synovium is hypertrophic or villous. Associated ligamentous lesions are described in Chapter 8.

POSTMENISCECTOMY PROBLEMS

Gear (1967) found that 10 years after meniscectomy 30 per cent of patients had disabling aching, stiffness or swelling of the joint. Dandy and Jackson (1975) have assessed clinically, radiologically and arthroscopically 174 knees with persisting problems. A retained fragment of meniscus was considered responsible for symptoms in 13 per cent of cases and lesions of the other meniscus were rare (5 per cent). However, early degenerative arthritis of the femoral condyle was present in 40 per cent of cases. The value of arthroscopic examination in reaching a diagnosis was highlighted by this article; for example, retained fragments of the posterior horn of the meniscus were found in only 10 per cent of their patients although a clinical diagnosis of three times this figure had been made. These authors also found that tears of the anterior cruciate or medial collateral ligament accounted for 10 per cent of the problems after meniscectomy; loose bodies were found in 2 per cent; and intra-articular adhesions were found in the region of the synovial scar in 9 per cent, in the suprapatellar pouch in 3 per cent and throughout the joint in 2 per cent.

Often the patient may complain of discomfort in, and around, the knee compartment which has been subjected to meniscectomy. This discomfort becomes most acute when sprinting and jumping. There may also be a dull ache along the related hamstring tendons. The cause of the knee discomfort is usually due to one of several factors, namely nipping of a still hypertrophic synovial frond, capsular or ligament strain due to the relative ligament laxity secondary to a loss of the meniscus, and 'pulling' of the hamstring tendons as they attempt to stabilize the knee. The part played by the 'bedding-in' process of the femoral condyle on the tibial plateau (with the relative increased loading over certain areas of the plateau which were formerly protected by the meniscus) is not fully evaluated. Certainly in animal experiments (Muckle and Minns, 1979) excessive shear forces following meniscectomy resulted in hyaline cartilage disruption within 8 weeks. Training on hard surfaces such as roads and concrete steps provokes knee pain and players should always attempt to carry out training on grass following the removal of a meniscus. If an effusion develops it should be aspirated and a compression bandage applied. Strains of the capsule, ligaments and hamstrings usually settle with rest, ultrasound and anti-inflammatories. Retained fragments, torn menisci and loose bodies need removal.

OSTEOARTHROSIS

This is a serious complication of meniscal damage. Tapper and Hoover (1969) found radiographic evidence of degeneration in 85 per cent of knees 10 years after meniscectomy. Jackson (1967) found radiographic

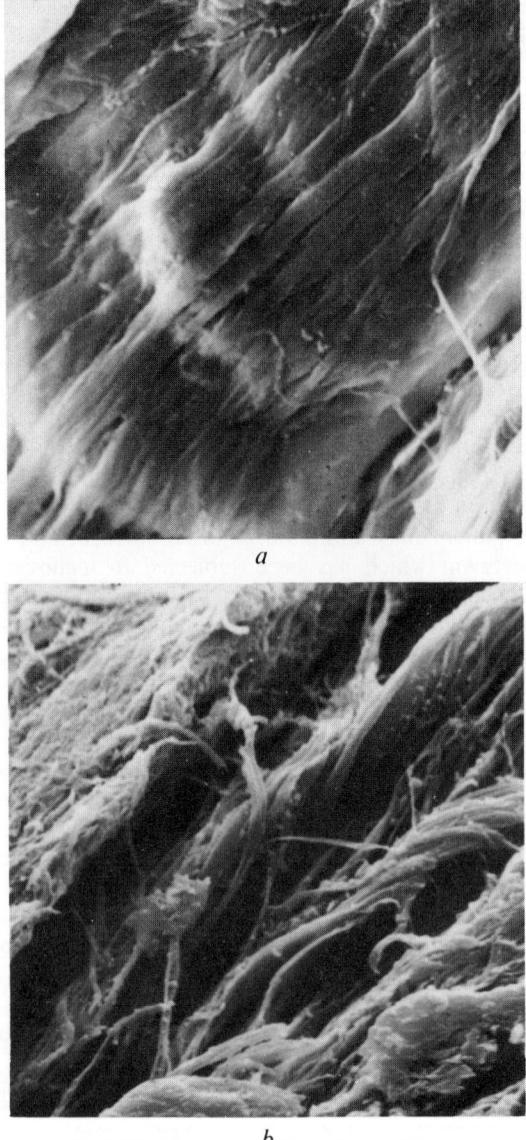

Fig. 28. Knee osteoarthrosis following meniscectomy. *a*, Normal human meniscus (scanning electron microscope) showing regularity of fibres (× 200). *b*, Disruption of fibres in a bucket-handle tear (× 200). *c*, Femoral hyaline cartilage erosions 8 weeks after meniscectomy (rabbit) (× 200). *d*, Bilateral osteoarthrosis most marked in the lateral compartment; lateral meniscectomy 6 years previously in a professional soccer player (Muckle and Minns, 1979; Muckle, 1980a).

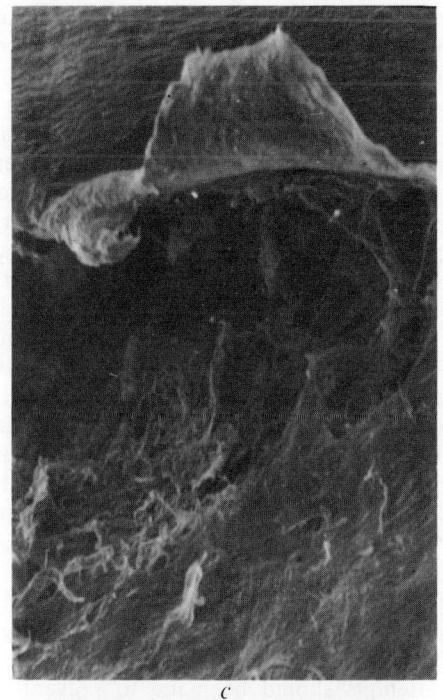

c

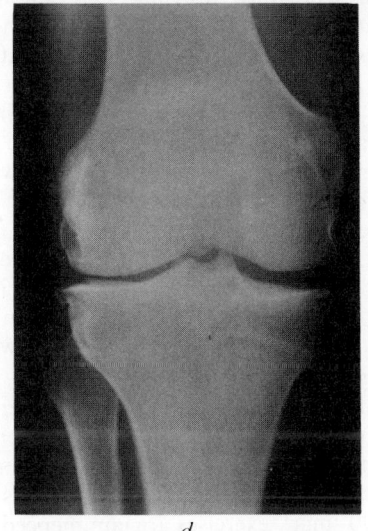

d

changes in 23 per cent (after 5 years) in the knee compartment without a meniscus, compared to 5 per cent in the other compartment where the meniscus had been retained.

Muckle (1980a) in a 12-year survey of 91 sportsmen found that all patients developed radiological changes of knee osteoarthrosis within 10 years following meniscectomy. Professional soccer players (50) showed the most severe changes and this was related to the increased frequency of knee trauma both before and after surgery. Another important contributory factor was knee ligament damage. Lax knees with an absent meniscus rapidly developed osteoarthritic changes (*Fig.* 28*d*).

Surprisingly, although radiological changes were present within 4 years or so of meniscectomy, rest pain was not a feature; although exercise-induced pain often terminated a sporting career. Patients with a lateral meniscectomy fared worse than with a medial. However, a delay between the original episode and surgery did not have an adverse effect unless there were frequent locking episodes. Partial meniscectomy patients showed less of the changes of osteoarthrosis compared to total meniscectomy.

POSTMENISCECTOMY REHABILITATION

A firm postoperative bandage is applied and straight-leg raising begins at 24 hours. In the presence of an effusion the quadriceps will be weakened and attempts should be made to prevent an effusion by careful haemostasis, pressure dressing and splintage, and if one develops, immediate aspiration. An athletic person should carry out 100 straight-leg raises and 200 static quadriceps contractions each day, the exercises being carried out in divided numbers (20 or so) for 5–10 min each hour. At 4–5 days the player is allowed up in a plaster cylinder which is removed at 10–14 days; otherwise it is the author's policy to keep the patient in bed for a 10-day period, allowing the soft-tissue reaction to settle and the wound to heal. During the first week of ambulation crutches are used, and the player does not carry his body weight on that leg. It has been the author's experience that too early weight-bearing and too vigorous knee mobilization in the initial stages of wound healing lead to a troublesome effusion which is usually bloodstained and may persist for 4–10 weeks (with the inevitable quadriceps wasting).

Thus the essential feature of the early postoperative period is to obtain soft-tissue healing and once this has been achieved and there is no joint swelling mobilization exercises can begin in earnest. Weight-bearing can commence with quarter squats, step-ups and cycling. Once flexion passes the 90° mark exercises are commenced against increasing resistance, with a weight applied to the foot and the knee flexed over a table. Discomfort during the exercises requires a cessation or a reduction in the applied weight. Pool therapy with the patient treading water or kicking in the water should be used during the third and fourth week. Then light training begins and sport is resumed at 6–12 weeks.

When the knee has regained good muscle power the athlete should begin with gentle running in a straight line; then in a figure-of-8 pattern, making large circles at first and gradually decreasing them in size. If this activity does not cause pain then running at speed can commence. However, sprinting has no place in the early rehabilitation after meniscectomy until muscle power is good and the player is proficient at jogging and turning.

Chapter 8

Ligamentous injuries in the knee

The assessment and classification of these injuries are the most complex and bewildering aspect of sports medicine; in order to overcome this confusion a picture will be progressively compiled from simple anatomical considerations.

STABILITY OF THE KNEE
Knee function must be considered under loaded and unloaded conditions. Under compressive loads the conformity of the condylar surfaces is the important factor in stabilizing the knee; however, the menisci by their wedge shape and variable concavity aid stability in the extended knee and up to 30° of flexion when only the lateral and posterior aspects are in contact. Beyond this point the ligaments restrict rotation whether or not the menisci are present. Under unloaded conditions the ligaments, menisci and capsule provided joint stability.

Soft-tissue Stabilizers
   a. Static stabilizers. The ligaments are not a group of isolated strands as depicted in anatomical preparations, each with a separate and distinct function; rather they operate as a cuff extending from slightly forwards of the midline both medially and laterally to the back of the knee.
   b. Dynamic stabilizers. If the ligaments and capsular fibres were to extend any farther forwards it would be impossible to flex the knee. Thus quadriceps muscle and its expansions provide dynamic stability. Posteriorly the hamstrings merge into the capsule in the same way.

For simplicity the capsule, ligaments and tendons can be divided into a *medial* and a *lateral compartment* (excluding the central cruciates) which in turn can be subdivided into thirds:

Anterior third: on both sides the ligaments are thin, loose and covered by the extensor retinaculum of the quadriceps.

Middle third: the capsular ligaments are strong and supported by the medial (tibial) collateral ligament medially and the iliotibial band laterally.

Posterior third: medially the capsule is thickened and receives the oblique popliteal expansion from the semimembranosus tendon; it is also augmented by the medial head of gastrocnemius. Laterally the lateral (fibular) collateral ligament, the arcuate ligament, an expansion from biceps femoris and the lateral head of gastrocnemius all provide extra stability.

Central Ligaments

The *anterior cruciate* extends from the tibia in front of the anterior spine (medial) to the lateral femoral condyle. When the knee is flexed to 90° this ligament is almost parallel to the tibial plateau. The major function is to prevent hyperextension and to act as a rotational guide during the screw-home mechanism of extension. The capsular ligaments prevent anterior rotatory instability but the anterior cruciate is an important secondary factor. Thus a tear of the anterior cruciate ligament associated with a tear of the medial or lateral capsular ligament will add to the severity of the anterior instability.

The *posterior cruciate* attached posteriorly on the tibia has a fan-shaped line of insertion on the medial femoral condyle. When the knee is extended, the posterior cruciate forms an angle of 30° to the horizontal and this angle changes only slightly during the full range of flexion. Both cruciate ligaments remain taut during movement and their cross-over point functions as the axis around which the knee moves both in flexion/extension and in rotation/gliding.

Instability (*Fig.* 29)

Instability of the knee is (*a*) straight or non-rotatory, (*b*) rotatory (simple or combined).

Straight instability. (1) Medial instability. (2) Lateral instability. (3) Posterior instability. (4) Anterior instability.

Rotatory instability. (1) Anteromedial instability. (2) Anterolateral instability. (3) Posterolateral instability. (4) Combined.

LIGAMENTOUS INJURIES
Sprain
This condition usually affects the collateral ligaments and chiefly the medial. There may be a small effusion or haemarthrosis which requires

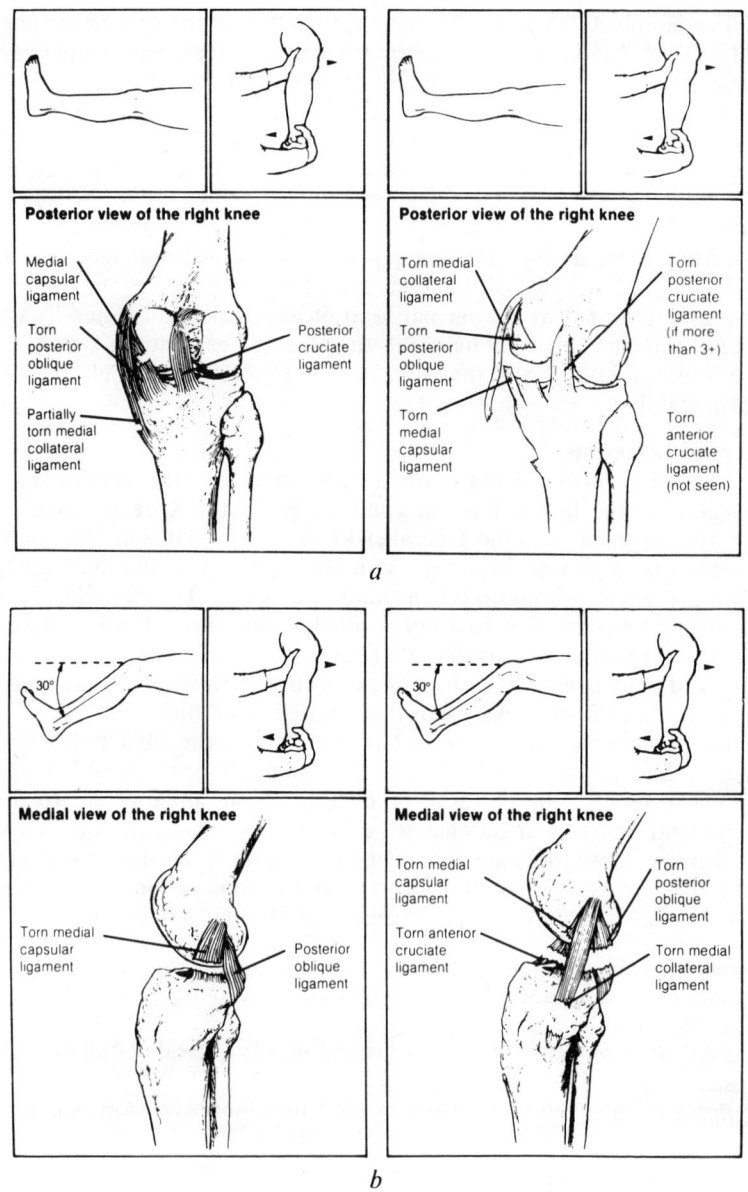

Fig. 29. *a*, Medial instability with the knee in extension. *b*, Medial instability with the knee at 30° of flexion. *c*, Lateral instability with the knee in extension. *d*, Lateral instability with the knee at 30° of flexion. *e*, Anterior instability at 15° of flexion. Posterior instability may be misdiagnosed as an anterior cruciate tear if the knee is not returned to a normal resting position before the Lachman test (Ritter and Gosling, 1980).

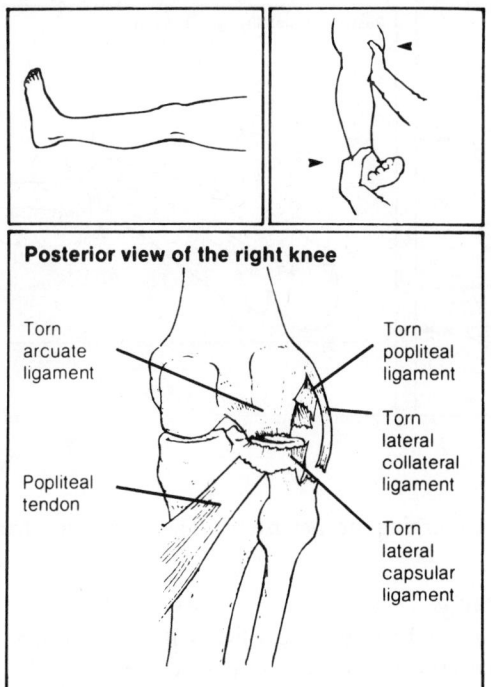

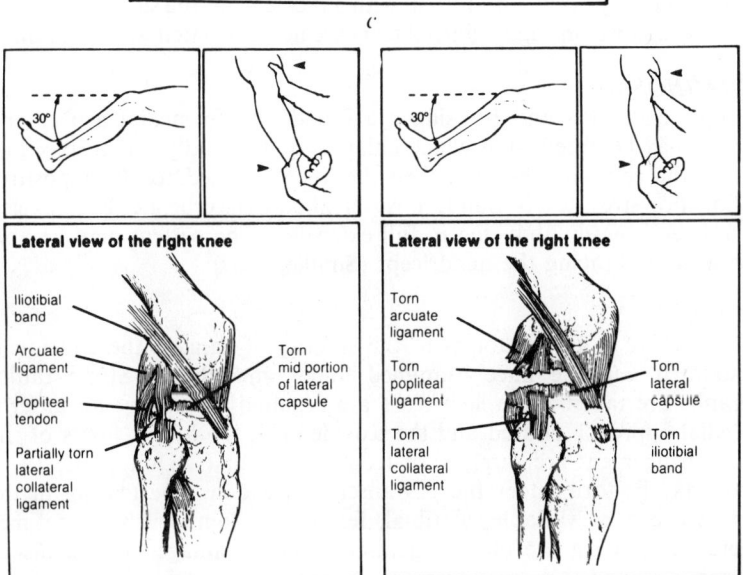

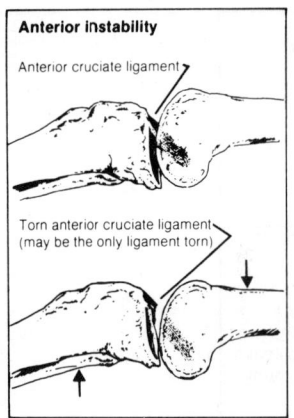
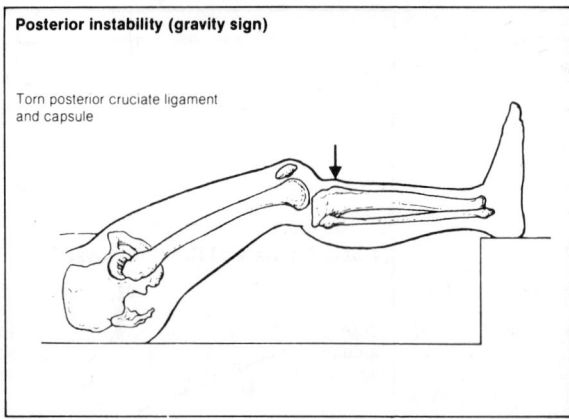

e

aspiration if enlarging or persistent. The treatment has been given in Chapter 4.

Medial Instability
A tear of the medial compartment ligaments leads to medial instability and associated cruciate damage adds to the severity of the instability. Such an injury occurs in football with a tackle from the side or when the scrum collapses in rugby. Partial tears are not associated with instability.

DIAGNOSIS
Local tenderness and bruising are found on the medial aspect and there may be an effusion which enlarges quite rapidly due to bleeding from the capsular vessels. When the knee is flexed to 30° a positive abduction stress test is found; however, should the cruciates be damaged the knee is easily abducted in full extension. The patient may be able to walk by bracing the quadriceps (Smillie, 1969).

TREATMENT
When there is any doubt as to the severity of damage the effusion is aspirated and the knee examined under anaesthesia. Stress radiographs are taken. Complete tears are repaired surgically: an anteromedial approach is used and the tear defined; the longer fibres of the medial ligament are rarely torn from the femur (O'Donoghue, 1973) but may be torn under the pes anserinus tendon. The tearing in the capsule can be variable, at tibial, femoral or joint levels, sometimes actually splitting the medial meniscus. When damaged the meniscus is removed and this procedure allows access to the posterior structures

which can be advanced and repaired. The medial ligament is completely repaired and the leg encased in a full plaster with slight flexion at the knee for 6 weeks.

Lateral Instability
Tears of the lateral compartment ligaments produce lateral instability, and, as in the case of medial instability, an associate cruciate damage (often posterior) adds to the severity of the injury. An adduction force alone or in combination with an internal rotation force is involved.

DIAGNOSIS
Pain and tenderness are located laterally and an effusion may be found. A positive adduction test is demonstrated in slight flexion of the knee; with associated cruciate damage this test is positive in extension.

TREATMENT
An anterolateral surgical approach is used: the iliotibial band must be explored to see that its attachment to the tibia is intact as well as its attachment to the femoral condyle through the intermuscular septum. The lateral ligament may be torn along its length, at the femoral insertion, or more commonly at the fibular attachment. It is repaired. The popliteus tendon and the biceps tendon may also be detached and require repair; while the lateral popliteal nerve is defined and protected. An associated cruciate injury also needs resuture. A plaster is worn for 6 weeks postoperatively with slight flexion at the knee. Reconstruction of the lateral ligament can be carried out using the split tendon of biceps femoris.

Posterior Instability
The posterior cruciate ligament is torn and laxity or rupture of the posterior ligamentous complex may be found.

DIAGNOSIS
A force is transmitted across the tibia (*Fig.* 30) from a falling player or tackle. Pain is felt behind the knee and tenderness and swelling are found in the popliteal space (this swelling is a haematoma). A positive drawer sign is found, the tibia moving abnormally backwards.

TREATMENT
When the tibial spine is avulsed, the small piece of bone is fixed with a pin or screw. If the posterior cruciate ligament is torn from the tibia, it can be secured with a mattress suture. If torn from its femoral attachment, the posterior cruciate can be fixed through a drill hole in the medial condyle of the femur at the front of the intercondylar notch. A tear in the middle portion is repaired by direct suturing.

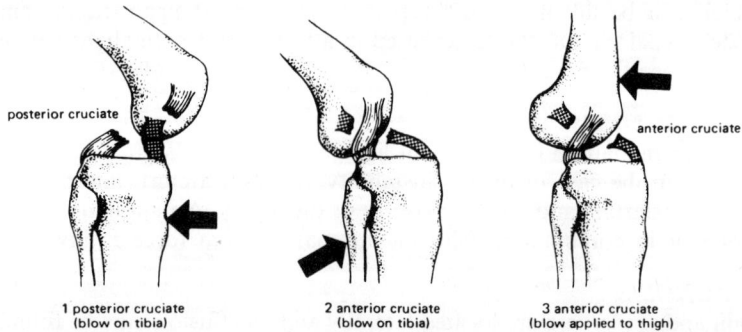

Fig. 30. The classic theory of cruciate damage by forces transmitted across either the tibial region or thigh. However, ligamentous damage in the knee is usually more complex and often involves the collateral ligaments and the posterior structures as well as the menisci.

However, O'Donoghue (1973) does not recommend primary reconstruction of the posterior cruciate, if badly torn, until a period of rehabilitation has determined whether other ligaments can compensate.

Anterior Instability
The anterior cruciate is damaged when a player falls from mid-air (basketball, heading at football) with the leg doubled-up beneath him. The force can be transmitted across the femur or from behind the tibia (*Fig.* 30).

DIAGNOSIS
Knee pain and swelling are found. The difficult diagnosis of a pure anterior cruciate ligament tear is made easier by the anterior drawer test in extension (Lachman test). With the knee in approximately 15° of flexion and the femur stabilized by a hand on the anterior aspect of the thigh, the tibia will demonstrate instability when moved anteroposteriorly. If the routine anterior drawer test is performed with the knee at 90° of flexion, the diagnosis can be missed.

TREATMENT
With ligamentous laxity a repair can be undertaken through a meniscectomy incision on the medial aspect of the knee, the detached anterior tibial spine being replaced and fixed. If the spine is not displaced, it can be held in place by a long-leg plaster with the knee in extension and operative intervention is not needed. Late reconstruction of the anterior cruciate has been described using the semitendinosus tendon (*Fig.* 31) (Cho, 1975). A plaster is worn for 6 weeks.

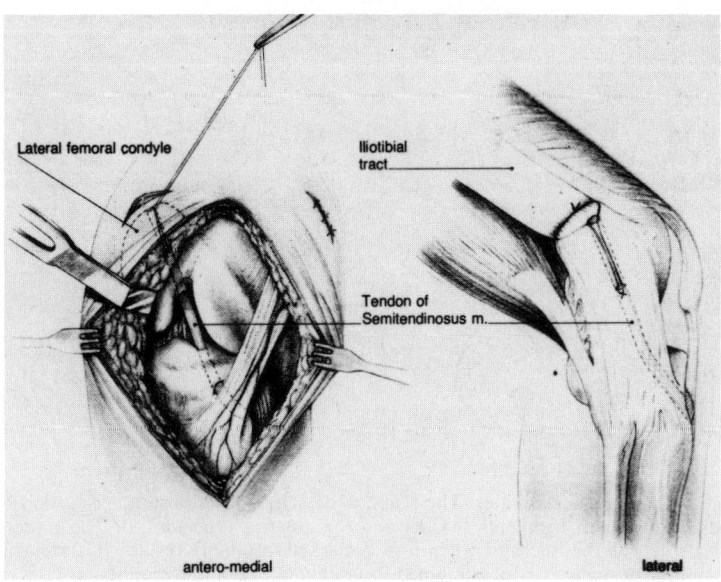

Fig. 31. Reconstruction of the anterior cruciate ligament using the semitendinosus tendon passed through a drill hole in the lateral femoral condyle. A guide wire is placed at the femoral insertion of the anterior cruciate ligament and the femoral hole (0·64 cm) is drilled from lateral to medial aspect using the guide (Cho, 1975).

ROTATORY INSTABILITY

If the posterior cruciate remains intact in the presence of other ligamentous damage then the tibia will rotate abnormally around this structure and rotatory instability results (*Fig.* 32).

Anteromedial Instability

The medial tibial condyle rotates abnormally forwards if the medial compartmental ligaments and posterior oblique ligament are torn. Such an injury is caused by a violent external rotation and abduction such as a tackle against the inner aspect of the leg which twists and throws the player laterally. At the same time the anterior cruciate and medial meniscus may be damaged.

DIAGNOSIS

The player has a painful swollen knee, but as the acute symptoms subside and training begins there is an inability to spring or turn rapidly, go up and down steps quickly or to carry out full squats. The player usually walks as if stiff-legged and may have difficulty in getting into and out of a car. He may have been subjected to a meniscectomy. A positive abduction test is found at 30° of flexion and if the foot is

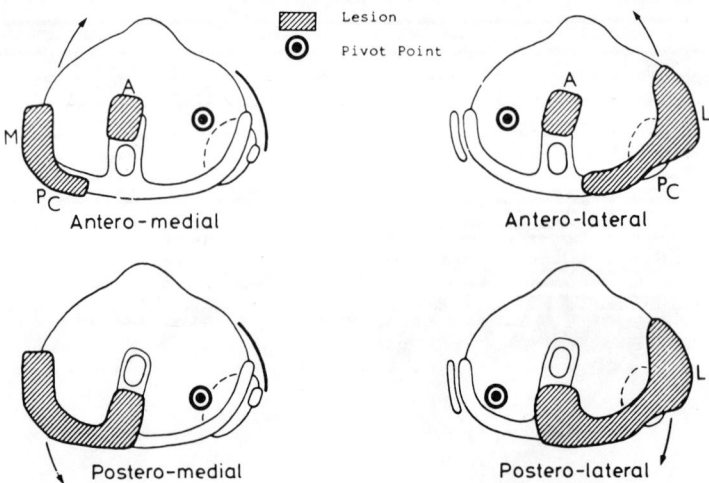

Fig. 32. Rotatory instabilities. The lesion is depicted in the posterior capsule (PC), medial and lateral ligaments (M, L) and the anterior cruciate (A). The posterior cruciate acts as the fulcrum; when torn a marked instability results. Posteromedial instability is usually part of combined instability (Dexel and Schreiber, 1979).

externally rotated a positive anterior drawer sign is elicited (i.e. the prominent medial tibial condyle can be pulled abnormally forward).

TREATMENT

The rotatory instability is best controlled surgically although a derotation brace has been described (Nicholas, 1973b). A pes anserinus transfer can be carried out; if damaged, the medial meniscus may be removed and the anterior cruciate repaired. The transfer involves the lower two-thirds of the conjoined tendon of sartorius, gracilis and semi-tendinosus muscles to a more proximal anterior insertion near the patellar tendon (Fig. 33) (Slocum and Larson, 1968). This enhances the power of internal rotation of the tibia and provides a sling support against the valgus thrust around the medial flare of the tibial condyle. Active muscle contraction is thus added to counteract the abnormal excessive external rotation. However, adequate posterior capsular stability is needed for this transplant to function satisfactorily because if there is posterior laxity the transplanted tendons will merely pull the tibia backwards rather than providing internal rotation. Postoperative immobilization is provided by a plaster cast with the knee at 30° of flexion for 6–8 weeks. Rehabilitation includes special exercises described in the article.

Nicholas (1973b) has described a five-one reconstruction for anteromedial instability of the knee. He points out that the anterior cruciate–medial posterior capsular complex injury can be associated with patellar subluxation or hypermobility. The surgical procedure is given in detail in this paper. The first step is to use a long medial lazy-S incision beginning at the adductor tubercle and swinging anteriorly across the anteromedial joint line and then turning to proceed distally and posteriorly. The pes anserinus tendon is divided vertically at the tibia in order to expose the distal part of the medial collateral ligament. The operator can see if this ligament is lax or scarred and also determine if the posteromedial capsular structures are slack. If inspection shows that the laxity is located above the level of the pes anserinus tendons then the medial ligament is detached with a flake of bone from the medial epicondyle and the interior of the knee exposed. The meniscus is removed to allow mobilization of the posterior capsule. Then the surgeon can visualize the large posterior capsular recess which is typical of a knee with anteromedial instability. The posterior part of the capsule is mobilized proximally behind the adductor tubercle and behind the flare of the medial femoral condyle. The leg is placed in full internal rotation and the tibia displaced posteriorly with the knee flexed between 30° and 60°. The upper part of the medial ligament is pulled upwards and backwards and reattached to the femoral condyle behind its original site. The reattached medial ligament should be taut enough to hold the leg in flexion and internal rotation. The posterior capsule is now pulled forwards and over the medial ligament and stitched to the anterior border of this ligament. The semimembranosus tendon which is brought forwards with the capsule is also fixed with several sutures (*Fig.* 33*b*). The posterior margin of the vastus medialis is mobilized and then sutured to the upper part of the advanced posterior portion of the capsule. Then the cut margin of the pes anserinus tendon is brought over the patellar ligament and stitched to the tibial crest, while posteriorly the turned-up edge of this tendon is sutured to the capsule (*Fig.* 33*b*). A plaster is applied with the limb held in full internal rotation and adduction and displaced backwards on the tibia, with the knee in 30° of flexion. Immobilization and non-weight-bearing are used for 6–8 weeks (*see* Nicholas, 1973b, for details).

Anterolateral Instability
This occurs when the leg is struck from behind or the side while the foot is plantigrade and the tibia is internally rotated and the stress placed laterally. A tear of the lateral compartment ensues and the anterior cruciate and lateral meniscus may be damaged.

DIAGNOSIS
The symptoms are as for anteromedial instability but the adduction stress test may be normal at 30°. However, there is a positive anterior

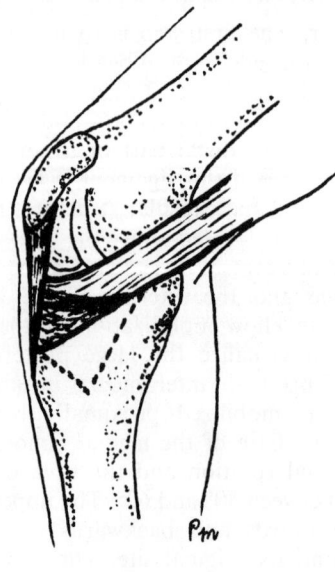

Fig. 33. *a*, The lower portion of the pes anserinus is sutured to the tibial tubercle and patellar tendon. The reflected lower border is then attached just below the upper end of the medial flare of the tibia anteriorly and to the upper margin of the sartorius medially and posteriorly (Slocum and Larson, 1968). *b*, Part of the Nicholas five-one operation. The five parts are as follows: meniscectomy, posterior and proximal advancement of the medial ligament, distal and forward advancement of the posteromedial capsule, advancement of the vastus medialis, and a pes anserinus transfer (Nicholas, 1973b). (*See opposite page*)

drawer test and lateral instability as shown by anterior subluxation of the lateral tibial plateau.

TREATMENT
See section *below* on combined instability.

Posterolateral Instability
This condition is the result of tears of the posterolateral structures and is caused by a blow against the anterior tibia with the leg externally rotated and in varus. The lateral ligament, popliteus and biceps tendon may be damaged.

DIAGNOSIS
The symptoms are as for anteromedial instability but the adduction stress test at 30° is positive and excess posterolateral rotation and a positive posterior drawer sign are found.

LIGAMENTOUS INJURIES IN THE KNEE 79

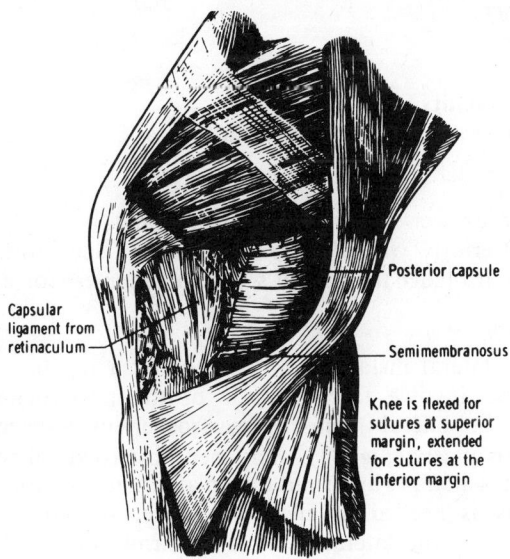

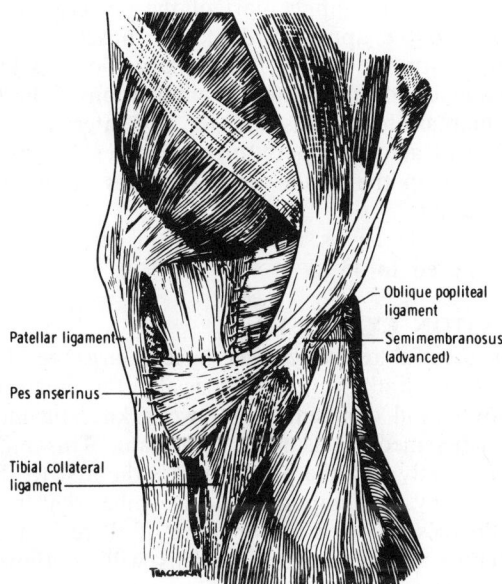

Fig. 33b

TREATMENT
See below.

Combined Instability
The result of tears of both medial and lateral compartments.

DIAGNOSIS
The anterior drawer sign is very positive and both tibial condyles subluxate anteriorly with the tibia in neutral. Such instabilities are uncommon but render the patient's knee functionless for most sports.

TREATMENT
All forms of lateral instability are treated by a repair of the lateral ligaments and involve fascial repair of the posterolateral corner, removal of the lateral meniscus, gastrocnemius advancement and biceps femoris plasty (*Fig*. 34); and when posterolateral rotatory subluxation is present a pes anserinus transplantation is performed. Lateral meniscectomy is needed to allow fascial repair and gastrocnemius advancement, for the lateral meniscus is firmly bound down to the posterior capsule and thus interferes with this reconstruction. Fascial repair tightens and advances the lower portion of the posterior capsule and the arcuate ligaments to the lateral ligaments. Gastrocnemius advancement tightens the upper part of the posterior capsule which is firmly bound to the upper third of this muscle; it also provides dynamic support for the posterolateral corner of the knee and decreases the tendency towards anterior subluxation of the tibia. Biceps femoris transplantation controls anterior and internal subluxation of the tibia and gives active support to the lateral side while decreasing the posterior pull on the fibular head. The pes anserinus transplant adds further stability.

Postoperatively the leg is immobilized in plaster for 6–8 weeks with the knee flexed to 45°.

REHABILITATION EXERCISES
The key to successful recovery after knee injuries resides in strong and healthy lower limb muscles, especially the quadriceps. Good quadriceps power will compensate for weak knee ligaments; in this respect the vastus medialis is most important. This muscle has its fibres inserted directly into the patella and is the first to show wasting after knee pathology. It is important to remember that it acts through the last few degrees of extension and that if there is a fixed flexion block or extensor lag the vastus medialis will continue to remain atrophic. The following exercises are instituted. The straight leg is raised to the count of 3, held for the same period and then lowered.

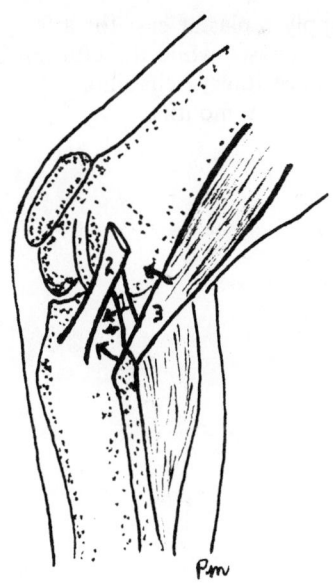

Fig. 34. The reconstruction operation for lateral instability of the knee using the lateral supporting structures. 1, The advancement of the lateral edge of the arcuate ligament and posterior capsule to the lateral capsule and fibular collateral ligament. 2, Lateral portion of the gastrocnemius tendon with its attached posterior capsule is brought forward and attached to the femur at a point anterior and superior to the proximal attachment of the fibular collateral ligament. 3, The biceps tendon is detached posteriorly from the fibula, its posterior two-thirds reflected, and the posterior margin sutured to the posterior edge of the iliotibial band (Slocum et al., 1973).

This is repeated in series of 10 to a maximum of 30. Whenever a series of 30 can be achieved easily weights are added to the foot in increments of 2 kg to a total of 10 kg. Daily progress should be charted. Straight-leg raising can be carried out on the back, lying on the unaffected side (abductor power) and face down (extensor power). Flexion exercises at the knee involve lying on the back and bending the knee by about 15° with the hip flexed to 40°. The knee is then extended and flexed to the same degree ten times. Weights can be added in 1–2 kg increments. This exercise builds up vastus medialis. The player can also sit with the leg hanging over a bench and the knee at a right angle, a spring system of weights with pulleys being used.

The success in knee rehabilitation is patience; each exercise must be mastered completely before the next one is undertaken. Pain and effusion require a reduction in activity and weights, and often it is advantageous to reapply a plaster cast for a few days and to concentrate on straight-leg exercises while the effusion and discomfort subside. After a major knee injury rehabilitation may take 3–6 months and sport is resumed at 6–9 months.

Chapter 9

Injuries to the tibia, ankle and foot

Such injuries are common in contact sports.

FRACTURES OF THE TIBIA AND FIBULA
Tibial Condyle Fractures
A fall from a height or a direct blow may fracture either or both tibial condyles. The fracture may be undisplaced and is commonly vertical in nature. Displaced fractures are frequently comminuted and small osteochondral fragments are liberated into the joint. In all cases the integrity of the ligaments must be assessed because the impaction of femoral condyle on to tibial condyle is often the result of a torn collateral ligament (*Fig.* 35).

DIAGNOSIS
The knee is swollen and painful, with angulation and ligamentous laxity.

TREATMENT
If the fracture is undisplaced the haemarthrosis is aspirated and a plaster applied for 6–8 weeks. Although displaced fractures can be reduced using traction and a tibial pin, surgery produces accurate reduction with internal screw fixation. Plaster immobilization is used for 4–6 weeks.

Because of the intra-articular disruption athletic ability usually falls due to knee stiffness and ligamentous weakness.

Fractures of the Fibular Shaft
These occur in footballers from a side tackle and are usually transverse and undisplaced. Such injuries need strapping or a below-knee plaster for 3 weeks. Sport can begin at 6 weeks depending on local discomfort.

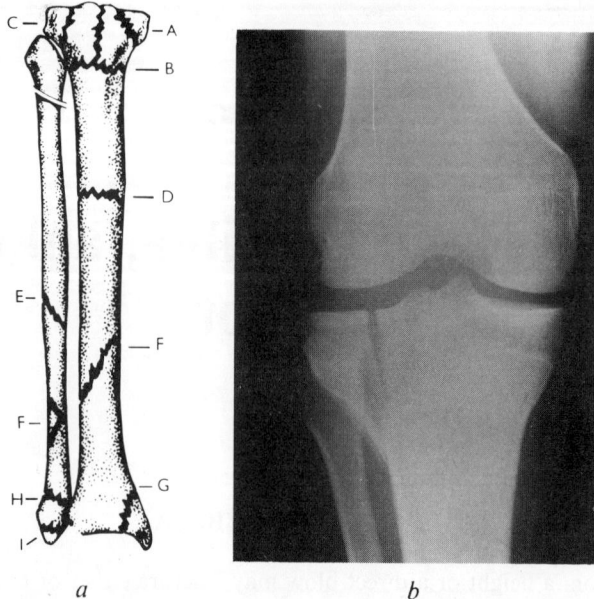

Fig. 35. *a*, Fractures of the tibia and fibula commonly found in athletes. A, Medial tibial plateau; B, T-shaped condylar; C, Lateral tibial plateau; D, Transverse midshaft; E, Fibular shaft; F, Spiral tibia and fibula; G, Medial malleolus; H, Lateral malleolus; I, Avulsion fracture. *b*, A fracture of the lateral tibial condyle caused by the lateral femoral condyle striking the tibia; such excessive movement can only occur with a rupture of the medial ligament.

Fractures of the Tibial Shaft

These may occur with or without a fibular fracture. A twisting force may cause a spiral fracture, a direct blow a transverse fracture (*Fig.* 35). These injuries are often compound.

DIAGNOSIS

Pain occurs over the fracture area and there is an inability to stand or move the leg.

TREATMENT

Undisplaced fractures require 6–8 weeks' non-weight-bearing in a full-leg plaster, with a further 2–4 weeks' partial weight-bearing while mobilizing the knee and ankle. Sport can begin at 6–9 months but refracture is common unless the player is proficient in all forms of stress exercises before undertaking full competition, especially football. Prolonged plaster immobilization leads to muscle atrophy, adhesions and joint stiffness; it is these soft-tissue complications which can mar future sporting performance. Clinical stability of the fracture is no proof that it will stand up to a strong tackle, the player must be rigorously tested with weight-training, running up and down steps, turning at speed and cross-country running before practice matches are allowed.

Displaced fractures require accurate reduction and if this cannot be achieved by closed methods due to the obliquity of the fragments or soft-tissue interposition then open reduction is performed. Compression plating is the treatment of choice and postoperatively the player can begin ankle movements once the pain and swelling have begun to subside, usually on the third day. If the fibula is not broken, it may have to be osteotomized to allow coaptation of the tibial fragments. Compound fractures require excision of the wound and antibiotics.

One of the problems with compression fixation is that little or no visible callus is produced. The presence of a large amount of external callus means that fixation is inadequate. The lack of callus on radiography means that the decision to remove the plate has to be arbitrary at 12–18 months; for too early a removal leads to refracture. Sport is resumed after a further 4–6 months; this delay allows the screw holes to fill with dense scar tissue and bone for the presence of screw holes reduces the strength of the bone to torsional loading by 30 per cent or more. Players should not participate with plates in situ because the plate can concentrate stresses and lead to a fracture below it or through a screw hole.

COMPLICATIONS

Arterial damage is sometimes severe and in any tibial fracture the anterior and posterior tibial pulses as well as the circulation in the toes must be examined. When the limb is badly swollen it is rested on a Thomas's splint and skeletal traction applied to the heel or lower tibia. Once the swelling has subsided then internal fixation or a plaster can be applied. Fasciotomy is rarely required but can be effective with gross compartmental oedema.

Swelling in either the anterior or posterior compartments may cause muscle fibrosis and this may lead to clawing of the toes, requiring tenotomy, tendon lengthening or arthrodesis. The dense fibrosis in the soleus and related muscles after a tibial fracture may impose a ban on first-class athletic performance despite apparent bony excellence on the radiographs.

Malunion is common and slight shortening is of little consequence providing that it is below 2 cm. Above this level the associated limp can hamper sporting ability and a shoe-raise must be provided. However, rotation and angular deformity are more disabling because the knee and ankle no longer move in the same plane and a corrective tibial osteotomy may be needed to restore normal function. Backward angulation is another major problem after tibial fractures because it is often accompanied by an equinus ankle and as the foot is forced upwards in walking the chance of refracture is increased and nonunion is common.

Delayed union is found in infected fractures, after gross displacement, with comminution and in double tibial fractures. Although conservative measures can be tried for 6–9 months a bone-grafting operation is usually needed at 4 months or so if the radiological changes of non-union are becoming apparent. Non-union may follow delayed union, especially if the plaster is discarded too soon or when the player has attempted to mobilize on a stiff ankle. Non-union is best treated by compression plating with bone chips.

Ankle stiffness is not uncommon after tibial fractures and along with oedema of the foot may persist for 6–9 months. Contrast bathing, pool exercises and a firm crêpe support are needed.

Stress Fractures

These may occur in the tibia or fibula and there is usually a history of progressive leg pain on running, relieved by rest (Devas, 1969). This condition is one form of shin soreness; rest, strapping or a plaster may be needed for 3–6 weeks (*Fig.* 36).

DISLOCATION OF THE KNEE

This is a severe injury producing gross ligamentous rupture and usually occurs in high-speed accidents although the author has seen a case sustained in a rugby tackle. Reduction and ligamentous repair are carried out but this injury usually terminates a sporting career.

DISLOCATION OF THE SUPERIOR TIBIOFIBULAR JOINT

A fall with the leg flexed and adducted with inversion at the ankle may dislocate this joint and pain may be referred along the lateral popliteal nerve. Reduction is achieved by flexing the knee and applying pressure on the fibular head (Muckle, 1973). Sport begins in 3–4 weeks.

ANKLE INJURIES

The ankle's movements in sport are complex and involve a shift of weight in the balanced action between trunk, hip, knee, ankle and foot. The ankle must maintain a balance on fixed surfaces such as ice or water, and absorb impact on uneven surfaces. In kicking the

INJURIES TO THE TIBIA, ANKLE AND FOOT

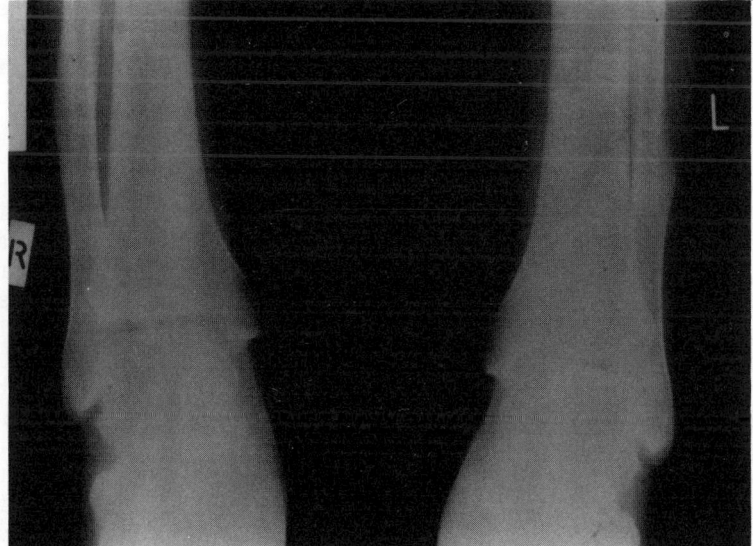

Fig. 36. Bilateral stress fractures of the fibula (long-distance runner).

ankle develops intense momentum to transfer from the body to the foot the kinetic energy to propel the ball. This synchronous movement requires a counterbalance thrust to the opposite ankle. The relationship between ankle and knee is important but complex; for example, in place kicking, the instep and entire forefoot twist on a fixed knee. With rotatory instability of the knee the rotational forces are transmitted to the foot via the ankle, producing a chronic sprain of the ankle ligaments.

In dorsiflexion the ankle mortise widens due to the fact that the head of the talus is broader anteriorly. Most commonly injuries to the ankle occur through forces applied to the mortise. Repeated stresses cause capsular osteophytes.

Sprains

Acute capsular sprains of the ankle are probably the commonest single type of sports injury. The classic injury is one of inversion and internal rotation which results in sprain of the lateral ligament complex. In the acute injury with local pain and swelling the treatment is by strapping or plaster depending on the severity of the problem. After 2–3 weeks the lesion resolves; more problematical is the less acute sprain which is often ignored because of the paucity of signs, the only gross physical sign being limitation of movement although careful inspection from behind shows filling of the sulcus on either side of the Achilles tendon due to posterior bulging of the joint. This injury requires immobilization as described above for it can be the precursor of a 'chronic sprained ankle'. (Emergency treatment of acute soft-tissue injury is described in Chapter 4.)

Chronic Sprained Ankle
When a sprain has become chronic the local tender area in the capsule is demarcated and treated with ultrasound, manipulation under local or general anaesthesia and local steroid injections. The ankle may have to be rested in plaster (below-knee) for 3–4 weeks, and a 'raise and float' may have to be applied to the heel of the shoe (usually 5 mm).

Spikes or studs which give excessive grip predispose to ankle problems and correct release bindings should be used by skiiers. Footballers who 'dangle' their foot into a tackle should have this fault rectified. Williams (1976) believes that ankle strapping may lead to local muscle atrophy and the build-up of stresses which can lead to substantial injury; however, many professional footballers routinely use ankle strapping especially after an ankle injury. Good muscle tone around the ankle is very important.

In any ankle injury a series of radiographs must be taken to exclude margin fractures, osteochondritis dissecans, osteophytes (footballer's ankle) and a calcaneonavicular bar (with peroneal spasm); a stress film is examined for ligamentous rupture.

Ligament Tears
Complete tears of the deltoid, calcaneofibular and tibiofibular ligaments are uncommon in isolation but usually accompany a fracture or dislocation. Repair of these ligaments should be carried out as the fracture is fixed internally. With a 'flake fracture' of the tips of the malleoli a stress film should be taken to investigate the integrity of the joint; when there is instability the torn ligaments should be repaired.

Lateral Ligament
In football the ankle is particularly vulnerable to sliding tackles or a clash of feet and the anterior fibres of the lateral ligament are torn with tenderness and swelling over the anterior aspect of the lateral malleolus. When the opposing player's boot comes through in a tackle from behind the posterior and middle fibres of the lateral ligament may be damaged.

DIAGNOSIS
There is local pain and swelling on the lateral aspect of the ankle

and severe bruising may be seen extending posteriorly to the Achilles region and on to the dorsum and sole of the foot. Instability may be shown by stress films and an arthrogram can be used in acute tears to show the extent of ligamentous damage (Nicholas, 1974).

TREATMENT

A walking cast is applied for 3–4 weeks. Nicholas (1974) does not advocate repair of the lateral ligament unless instability is present in two planes and an arthrogram shows major damage. At surgery the joint is cleared of clotted blood and the shredded ligaments opposed with dexon. The foot is placed in slight valgus initially to take the strain off the suture line. A plaster is worn for 3–4 weeks and mobilization exercises should be designed to regain full inversion before competition is resumed, especially football.

Surgery is recommended in cases of chronic recurrent instability. Good et al. (1975) have devised a simple operation for reconstruction of the lateral ligament using the peroneus brevis tendon (*Fig.* 37). Nicholas (1974) advocates the Elmslie operation in which the peroneus brevis tendon is split and brought through an anteroposterior drill hole in the fibula and across the calcaneus in a vertical direction

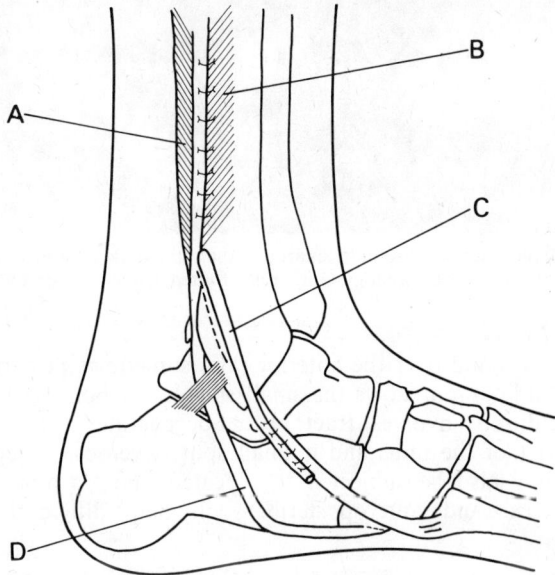

Fig. 37. Reconstruction of the lateral ligament of the ankle using the peroneus brevis tendon (C) passed through a hole drilled in the fibula and sutured back on itself. A is the peroneus longus muscle belly, B the peroneus brevis muscle belly sutured to (D) the peroneus longus tendon (Good et al., 1975).

through the subtalar region and back into the cuboid. There is thus an anterior talofibular as well as a fibulocalcaneal component.

Footballer's Ankle
This condition is not an osteoarthrosis of the ankle joint; examination of the joint surface at surgery usually reveals no damage to the hyaline cartilage. However, numerous small capsular tears cause marginal osteophytes which may impinge on the neck of the talus during 'dead-ball kicking'. This leads to discomfort on shooting and later a dull pain (*Fig.* 38).

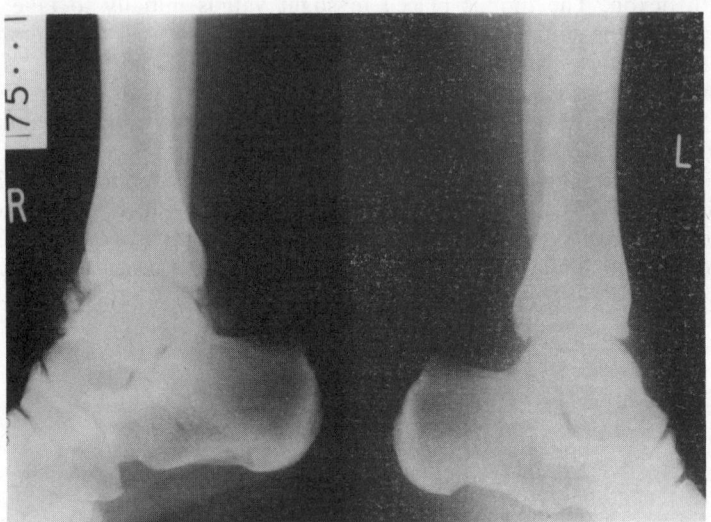

Fig. 38. Footballer's ankle—osteophytes around the right ankle joint in a professional soccer player (this man was predominantly right-footed as the radiographs indicate).

DIAGNOSIS
Tenderness is found over the anterior (and sometimes posterior) joint line and a radiograph shows the small spicules of bone. A somewhat similar condition involves fracture or degenerate changes in the posterior part of the talus and a small spur develops. A separate os trigonum may also be subjected to repeated minor trauma. Radiographs (lateral and anteroposterior) will help differentiate these conditions.

TREATMENT
In the early stages kicking should be reduced and short-wave diathermy given. Surgery is needed when the spicules have become prominent or fractured, and when loose bodies are present.

Ankle Fractures

These may occur with or without a dislocation or subluxation (as in the typical Pott's fracture). Usually the foot is anchored to the ground while the momentum of the body continues forwards. The most important forces are external rotation and either abduction or adduction of the ankle.

DIAGNOSIS
The ankle is swollen and painful and the deformity is obvious.

TREATMENT
Conservative Treatment
Conservative treatment and plaster immobilization for 6–12 weeks can be used when there is little or no displacement or when there has been a very accurate reduction. The foot is placed at a right angle to the leg and must be in a neutral position (i.e. not in varus or valgus).

Surgery
This is required to ensure perfect reduction and to maintain it in unstable fractures, to remove soft tissues which are intervening in the fracture line (e.g. tibialis posterior tendon) and to repair the ligamentous damage (*Fig. 39*).

Müller et al. (1970) have outlined the essential features of surgery in ankle fractures. They point out that the ankle mortise depends on the correct length of the fibula and the integrity of the anterior and posterior tibiofibular ligaments. The fibula with its taut elastic attachment to the tibia takes absolute priority over the medial malleolus. Damage to the tibiofibular syndesmosis can be deduced from the level of the fracture. A fracture of the fibula at the level of the ankle joint or below this is never associated with a lesion of the syndesmosis. By contrast, a fracture of the fibula above this level is always associated with a lesion of either the anterior or the posterior tibiofibular ligament (Weber, 1966). Besides injury to the malleoli and ligaments there may be avulsion, shear osteochondral or chondral fractures of the talus, and these may produce loose fragments in the joint.

Internal fixation of the lateral malleolus is carried out with one or two screws or a small plate. Torn ligaments are repaired and stabilized with screws if necessary (*Fig. 40*). If the interosseous membrane has been torn, in addition to the repair, the syndesmosis is protected by further stabilization of the fibula. The medial malleolus, posterior malleolus and deltoid ligament are repaired and stabilized using small screws or tension band wiring.

Postoperatively the leg is elevated for 4–5 days and rested in a plaster splint with the foot at 90°. After 48 hours dorsiflexion exercises

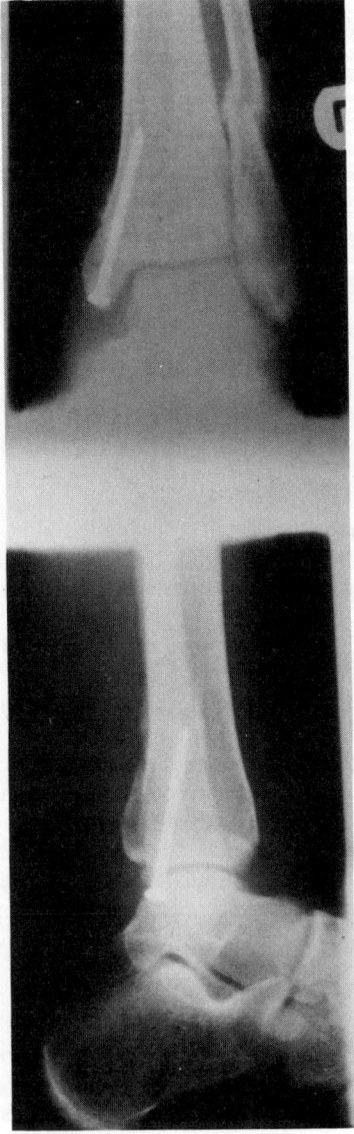

Fig. 39. Internal fixation of the medial malleolus.

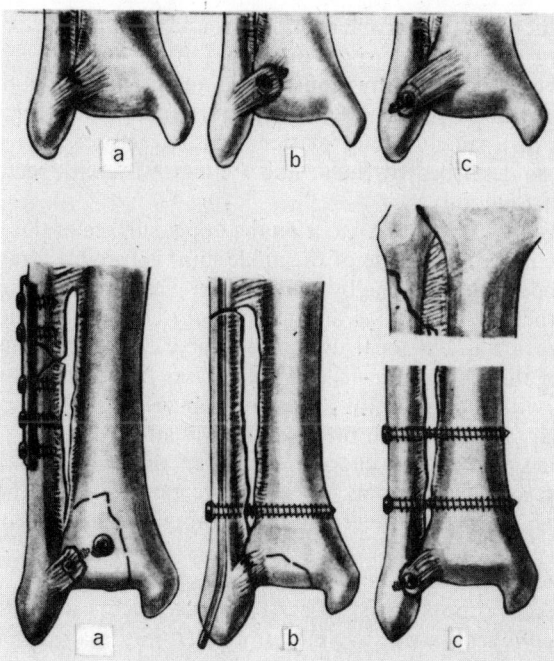

Fig. 40. Stabilization of the tibiofibular syndesmosis. *Upper*: The anterior tibiofibular ligament can be torn in its mid-point (*a*); tibial insertion (*b*); or fibular insertion (*c*). *Lower*: The syndesmosis, once repaired, is protected in three different ways. A small semitubular plate can be employed (*a*); intramedullary nailing of the fibula with a non-lagged screw (*b*); or when the whole interosseous membrane has been disrupted (e.g. with a fracture of the fibular neck) one or two position screws are used (*c*). (After Müller et al., 1970.)

are commenced. At 14 days partial weight-bearing is begun in a below-knee plaster if the original fixation was less than excellent; otherwise a removable splint can be used. The plaster is worn for 6–8 weeks. At the end of this period the screws etc. can be removed under local anaesthesia. Sport begins at 4–6 months.

FOOT FRACTURES

Fractures of the talus are rare and are due to considerable violence. There may be a fracture-dislocation but a frank dislocation is sometimes found (Kenwright and Taylor, 1970). Displaced fractures need urgent reduction in order to avoid early skin necrosis and late avascular changes in the talus. The circulation in the foot should be monitored. A below-knee plaster is applied after reduction and worn for 6 weeks.

Calcaneal fractures are complex and when they involve the subtalar joint produce the late problems of pain and swelling especially when the athlete runs on hard or uneven ground. A persistent heel discomfort may also be found for many months after an undisplaced body fracture. Such undisplaced fractures require a crêpe bandage with thick wool for 4–6 weeks or a snugly-fitting plaster. Crush fractures may need open reduction as described by Soeur and Remy (1975) with reconstruction of the subtalar joint.

An avulsion fracture can occur on the upper surface of the neck of the talus if the anterior capsule of the ankle joint is forcibly stretched as in contact sports such as rugby and soccer. Similarly the interosseous ligament (between the talus and calcaneum) can be stretched or torn resulting in a marked local discomfort especially during inversion or eversion of the calcaneum. In persistent cases the interosseous canal is infiltrated with local steroids and a local anaesthetic. Manipulation of the subtalar joint may also break down any adhesions.

Crush injuries of the cuboid, navicular or cuneiform bones are uncommon and if symptoms are severe warrant a below-knee plaster-of-Paris for 2–3 weeks; otherwise firm strapping can be used.

SEVER'S DISEASE
Sever's disease (apophysitis) (*Fig.* 41) usually occurs in boys of about 9–10 years of age. It is due to a mild traction injury; pain and tenderness are localized to the insertion of the Achilles tendon. Sometimes there is an increased density and fragmentation of the apophysis.

Treatment
This is a self-limiting condition. Rest from sport for 1–3 months, with a plaster when the heel is very swollen.

After a blow to the heel, as in soccer, a localized heel haematoma can simulate Sever's disease, and occasionally an infection of the calcaneum may develop. When the heel is quite tender and swollen a precautionary ESR should be taken. Bursitis just above the insertion of the Achilles tendon may result from ill-fitting footwear and has to be differentiated.

Apart from fractures and Sever's disease, calcaneal pain may be due to a localized infection or calcaneal spur (in plantar fasciitis). Acute plantar fasciitis may have a rheumatological (Reiter's syndrome) or infective (e.g. gonorrhoea) basis and the appropriate tests should be made.

PAINFUL TARSUS
In children, pain in the mid-tarsal region is rare; one cause is Köhler's disease (osteochondritis of the navicular). The bony nucleus of the navicular becomes dense and fragmented. A comparable condition occasionally develops in middle-aged women (Brailsford's disease). In

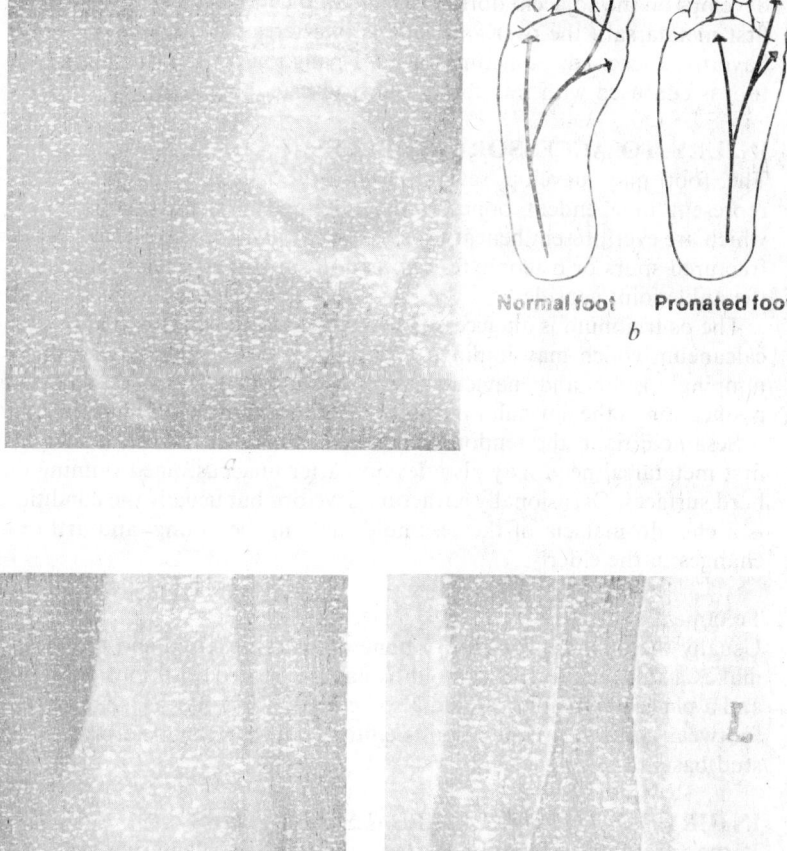

Fig. 41. *a*, Sever's disease in a young female gymnast (9 years). *b*, The pronated foot which may accompany tibial torsion, genu valgus and familial joint laxity (a common cause of apparent flat foot, when a normal arch occurs on standing on tip-toes). *c*, Peaking of the medial malleolus in a soccer player due to deltoid ligament ossification. *d*, Pain around the ankle. 1, Os trigonum injury, 2, Osteophyte fracture, 3, Flake fracture talus, 4, Interosseous ligament strain, 5, Calcaneonavicular bar (spasmodic flat foot).

young adults, especially if the arch is high, a ridge of bone sometimes develops on the adjacent dorsal surfaces of the medial cuneiform and the first metatarsal ('the overbone'). This interferes with kicking and may have to be excised. Sometimes a hard ganglion on the dorsum of the foot is confused with this condition. It also requires removal.

INJURY TO ACCESSORY OSSICLES

The foot may develop several accessory ossicles; sometimes they represent independent bones (most obvious by the sesamoid bones which are ever present beneath the first metatarsal head) or they may be fractured spurs or osteophytes retained in soft-tissue structures such as the ankle joint capsule.

The os trigonum is an accessory bone behind the talus and above the calcaneum which may impinge on the talus during plantar flexion of jumping. Talar and navicular spurs, and independent centres of ossification in the navicular may also be nipped during joint movements.

Sesamoiditis in the tendon of flexor hallucis where it lies under the first metatarsal head may also develop after unaccustomed running on hard surfaces. Occasionally a fracture develops but usually the condition is a chondromalacia of the sesamoid facet in the young, and arthritic changes in the elderly.

Treatment

Usually the offending accessory bone or spur is excised and the player makes a full recovery. Sesamoiditis can be treated with local steroids, and a plaster. Attention should also be paid to the internal shape of the footwear and any pressure points eliminated, for example a protruding stud base.

INJURY TO THE METATARSALS AND TOES

If the forefoot is violently twisted, abducted or plantarflexed, tarso-metatarsal dislocation may occur. The first metatarsal is either dislocated or fractured near its base. Such injuries occur with horse-riding and motorcycle accidents, especially if the foot is trapped by a stirrup or bar. This is a serious injury and the circulation of the foot may be impaired. Thus reduction is urgent and maintained by a padded split-plaster. The plaster is retained for 3 weeks.

Any of the toes or metatarsal bones may be damaged by a crushing injury. Generally the terminal phalanx or the metatarsal necks fracture. Isolated metatarsal fractures rarely displace and can be treated by a firm strapping support. The injured toe can be strapped to its neighbour for 10 days, but kicking may be painful for several weeks. The great toe is a special problem because discomfort may persist for several months after a fracture and any associated stiffness of the metatarsophalangeal joint or the phalangeal joints causes some disability during the 'toe-off' phase' of sprinting. In all foot injuries malunion may result in only minimal disability, angulation can produce a bone prominence which causes pressure areas in the sole or friction against shoes and boots.

AVULSION INJURY
Forced inversion of the foot may cause an avulsion injury of the fifth metatarsal base. In children the styloid epiphysis feels tender.

Treatment
Strapping and early mobility are encouraged. However, normal inversion which stretches the peroneus brevis during walking sometimes exacerbates the pain and thus a plaster is required for 2 weeks.

MARCH FRACTURE
In young athletes, especially after prolonged road work, the foot becomes painful and a tender lump may be felt just midshaft of the metatarsal bone. Usually the second metatarsal is affected. In the early stages a fine crack is seen, later a large mass of callus forms.

Treatment
Rest from sport until symptoms subside, usually 3–4 weeks. Correct attention to good soles on the running shoes, while training on grass surfaces prevents recurrence.

SUBUNGUAL PAIN
A player may tread on an opponent's toes and produce a subungual haematoma which should be released with a sterile needle. An associated fractured terminal phalanx must be excluded. Deformity of the toe nail may indicate a subungual exostosis which should be removed surgically. This usually requires avulsion of the toe nail. A glomus tumour is a rare cause of subungual pain. A recurrent ingrowing toe nail needs removal (Zadik, 1950).

METATARSAL AND FOREFOOT PAIN
An apparent flattening of the longitudinal arch of the foot is frequently found in children, but this is only an expression of generalized ligamentous laxity. Standing on tip-toes reproduces the normal arch. Occasionally shoe pads are needed but generally no treatment is required and the arch resumes its normal configuration during adolescence. In elderly athletes a fixed fallen transverse arch occurs, callosities developing beneath the metatarsal heads. Pads are effective in the early stages but a metatarsal osteotomy may be needed, the second to fifth metatarsal necks being divided and the arch reformed with

either plaster-of-Paris for 4 weeks or early mobilization with crêpe strapping.
Slight flattening of the longitudinal arch can cause plantar fascial strain, nipping of the intertransverse ligaments, bursitis between the metatarsal heads, and neuroma formation (Morton's neuroma). Clawing of the toes becomes a secondary feature following a fallen transverse arch. Deviation of the hallux may also be found (hallux valgus). Hallux rigidus occurs in some athletes, especially if the first metatarsal is short. Avulsion of the flexor accessories from the calcaneum is a rare injury having been found in a soccer player after an attempted jump was blocked by an opponent's foot on his boot.

Treatment
This follows conventional orthopaedic teaching. Intrinsic foot exercises can be used for foot strain. Surgery is needed in Morton's neuroma, hallux valgus and hallux rigidus. In older athletes a Keller's arthroplasty may suffice but often this procedure simply transfers weight bearing to the second and third metatarsal heads with later problems of pain, callosities and clawed toes. An osteotomy of the first metatarsal (such as an oblique osteotomy or a Mitchell's procedure) can be used in young athletes with hallux valgus. Arthrodesis of the great toe can be used for hallux rigidus; Silastic implants risk infection and implant failure in many sportsmen. Well-fitting running shoes, plimsoles or boots prevent undue crowding of the transverse arch.

THE PRONATED FOOT
The pronated foot (*Fig.* 41*b*) is one of the more common foot disorders suffered by athletes, usually due to excessive running. The pronated foot disrupts the normal path of weight-bearing and causes exaggerated internal rotation of the leg. Flattening of the longitudinal arch, with tenderness of the plantar fascia, medial ankle ligaments and posterior tibial tendon, occurs. Spasm follows in the peroneal muscles and the interosseous ligament becomes stretched. Finally the forefoot spreads out and the metatarsal heads become painful. In the mildly pronated foot there is 4–6° of calcaneus valgus, a severe deformity of 12° may sometimes be found.

Treatment
Ice massage, cold whirlpool and galvanic muscle stimulation or transcutaneous nerve stimulation are used. Anti-inflammatory agents are given. Arch supports or orthotic devices supplied by a podiatrist can be used. Some exercises help to control pronation. Toe rises and Achilles tendon stretching exercises strengthen the calf muscles; the toes should be exercised by picking up small objects (e.g. marbles).

Finally, the player should be encouraged to walk with a slight toe-in gait and an exaggerated spring in pushing off.

GAIT

Variations in the angle of gait are observed in various sports (*Fig.* 42), this angle being formed by the line of progression and the footstrike position. A wide based gait is desired for stability. However, as a rugby player breaks away from a defensive position he assumes a more upright position, and as his speed increases, his base of gait becomes more narrow until it reaches zero i.e. the weight-bearing foot lands

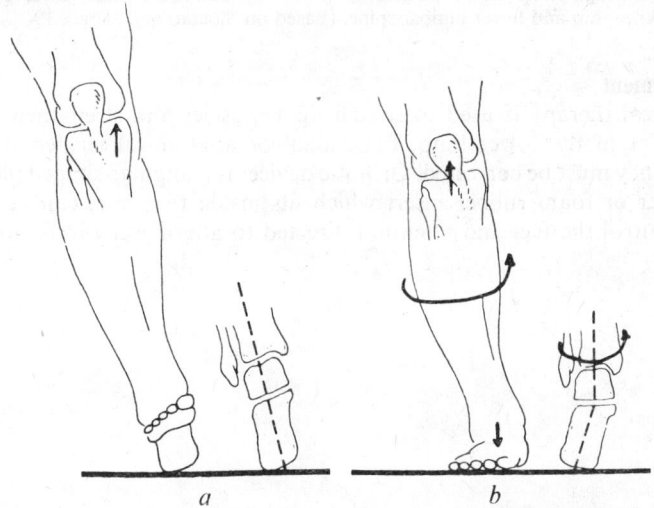

Fig. 42. *a*, The varus gait with stresses on the lateral ligament complex of the ankle and the medial compartment in the knee. *b*, The valgus gait with pronation of the foot, associated spreading of the foot arches, tibial torsion, and rotatory stresses in the knee and ankle. (Based on Subotnick, 1975.)

under the centre of gravity (*Fig.* 43). Thus the body above the foot is well balanced. However, variations in gait and imbalance can lead to lower limb overuse injuries, especially in the ankle and foot. A slight limb length discrepancy results in an overstride with the shorter leg; if there is 1 cm or more shortening the runner may externally rotate the short leg and foot for additional lateral stability. Thus anterior shin-splints may occur. Tibial torsion, genu varus or valgus may also concentrate forces so that stress fractures occur in the tibia, femoral neck or lumbar spine.

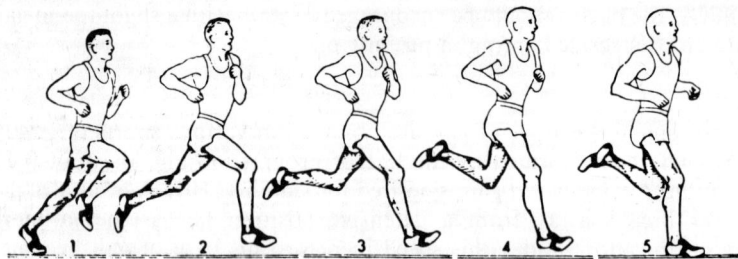

Fig. 43. The phases in running result in stresses as depicted. In (1) the Achilles tendon and the forefoot are stressed; in (3) the hamstrings are stretched during the follow-through phase; in (5) the contact with the ground causes stress loading of the tibia, knee, hip and lower lumbar spine. (Based on Slocum and James, 1968.)

Treatment

Physical therapy is used to stretch tight muscles and strengthen weak muscles in the lower limb. Functional or anatomical leg length discrepancy must be corrected. Orthotic devices (an angular-shaped plastic, leather or foam rubber insert which fits inside the shoe) can be used to control the feet and attention directed to altering any imbalance in style.

Chapter 10

Shoulder and upper limb injuries

These injuries account for one-fifth of all sports injuries; they can be sports specific such as 'javelin elbow' or 'baseball finger', or non-specific such as acromioclavicular dislocation or a supracondylar fracture. It is also worth recalling that epiphysial damage may be produced by either direct trauma (*Fig.* 44) or by repeated trauma as exemplified by damage to the elbow epiphysis as a result of throwing (known in the United States as 'little league arm'). A negative radiograph in a child does not exclude epiphysial damage. Any throwing sport can also cause a stress fracture of the humerus (Devas, 1969).

ACROMIOCLAVICULAR DISLOCATION
This injury is usually produced by a fall on the tip of the shoulder but may occur when the shoulders are pinned to the floor in wrestling. Reduction is difficult to maintain because of the obliquity of the articular facets. It is important to remember that in subluxation the superior and inferior capsule are torn but that the main stabilizing ligament, the coracoclavicular ligament, remains intact. Thus, conservative measures such as a looped adhesive strapping over the shoulder and around the elbow or even a broad arm sling are effective and the player can resume activity after 2–3 weeks.

In a dislocation (*Fig.* 45) the coracoclavicular ligament is ruptured and this permits wide separation of the two fragments. Clinical appearances show an elevation of the outer aspect of the clavicle but this may be masked by oedema. Conservative treatment is usually by adhesive loop strapping (as for subluxation), a webbing harness or a plaster spica—for 3–4 weeks (Bearden et al., 1973).

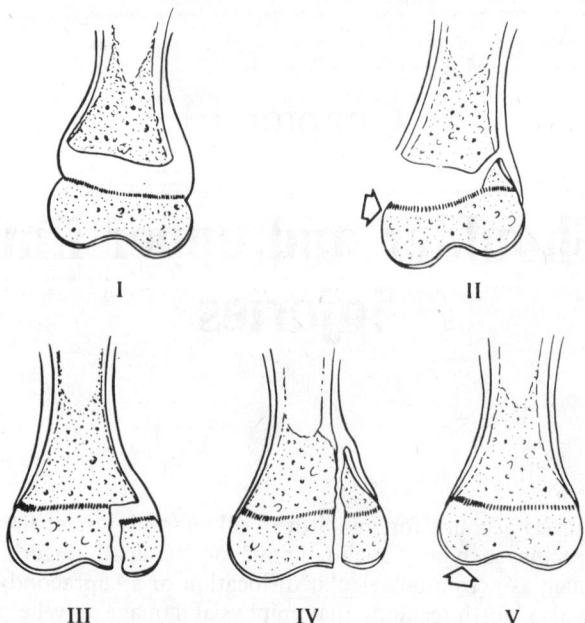

Fig. 44. Classification of epiphysial fractures. Type I fractures separate through the epiphysial plate; Type II fractures also carry a triangle from the metaphysis; Type III fractures have a vertical element in the epiphysis; Type IV fractures traverse the epiphysis, plate and metaphysis; Type V fractures are crush injuries to the epiphysial plate (Salter and Harris, 1963).

However, Scott and Orr (1973) reported that with conservative treatment of a dislocation 60 per cent had residual deformity and half of these patients had symptoms referable to the injured joint. Several surgical measures are available. The simplest method is by Kirschner wire fixation after reduction; this can be done with a percutaneous technique and the shoulder immobilized with plaster or an extensive looped strapping to shoulder and upper chest. However, this technique ignores the coracoclavicular ligament and open reduction with repair is probably better, the bones being fixed with a Kirschner wire, screw or wire loop. Behling (1973) recommends clavicle/coracoid fixation with a lag screw which is removed under local anaesthesia 6 weeks later; he states that repair of the ligament is not necessary. A sling is worn and gentle shoulder mobilization carried out. After surgery sport can begin in 3 months.

The Bailey procedure is more involved and requires detachment of the distal portion of the coracoid process with the conjoined tendon of the short head of biceps and coracobrachialis and fixation of the bony process plus tendons to the outer part of the clavicle. Muscle forces hold the clavicle in position and mobilization of the shoulder begins at 6–8 weeks. Whereas simple fixation with wires or screws is

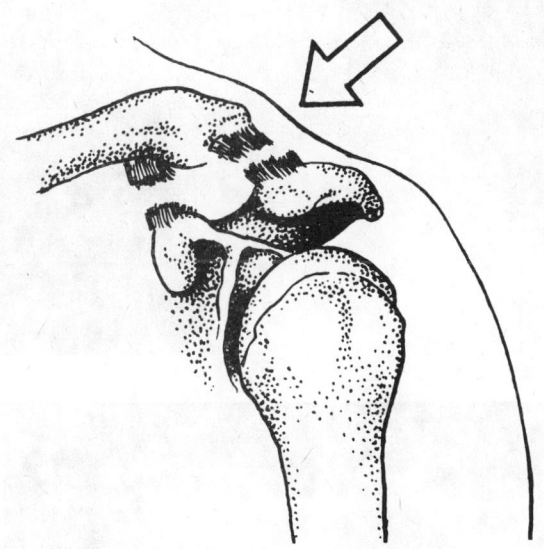

Fig. 45. Dislocation of the acromioclavicular joint.

effective in contact sports such as rugby and football, the Bailey procedure has been advocated in sports requiring mobility plus stability such as throwing events, basketball, etc.

Some injuries are missed or fail to respond to conservative measures and the athlete may present months or years later with a painful subluxation or dislocation. However, the author has known several sportsmen compete up to international level with chronic subluxation and a painless shoulder. In the presence of a painful, old injury the outer end of the clavicle can be excised (Muckle, 1972a).

SHOULDER DISLOCATION
Dislocation of the shoulder is a problem in sports injuries because recurrence is not uncommon in fit, young athletes who return to stressing their shoulders and surgery necessarily imposes a restriction   shoulder mobility, often with a lowering of sporting performance.

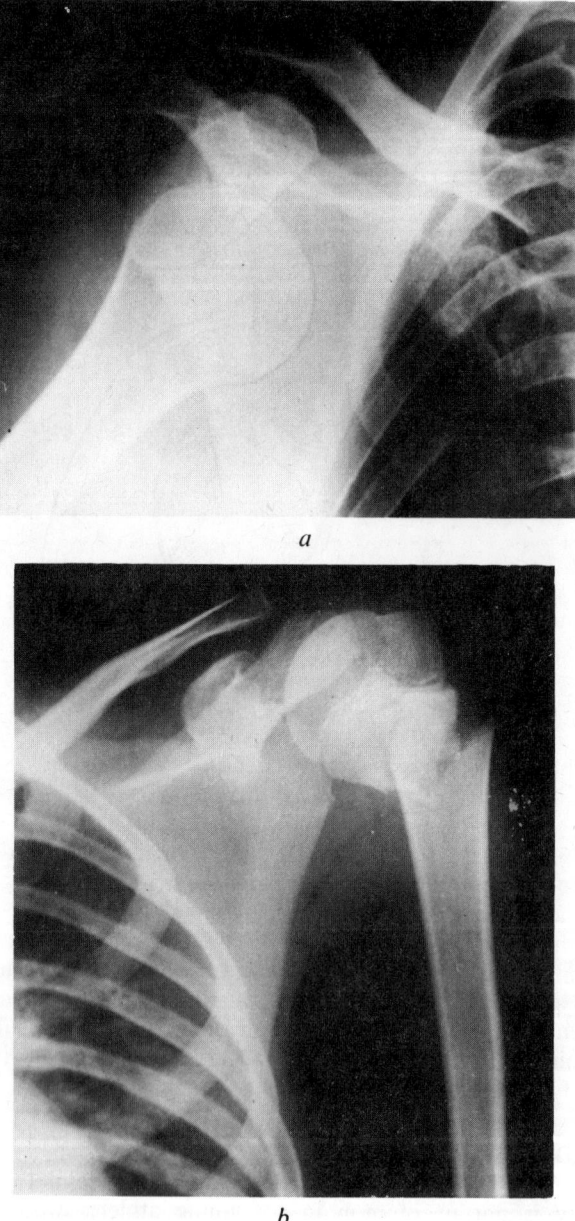

Fig. 46. *a*, A dislocation of the shoulder (anterior) can be confused clinically with *b*, a fracture of the upper humerus. Hence the need for radiological confirmation in all cases of suspected dislocation.

ANTERIOR DISLOCATION

By far the greatest number of shoulder dislocations are anterior (*Figs.* 46 and 47), being common in high jumpers and water polo, wrestling, judo, football and rugby players. It occurs with an extension force to an abducted, externally rotated arm as in a 'hand-off' at rugby.

Diagnosis

There is a sickly shoulder pain with muscle spasm and the resulting deformity due to the prominent humeral head is obvious—the arm being supported in a slightly abducted position.

Treatment

Although it is common practice to reduce the dislocation immediately it should not be forgotten that an associated fracture of the humeral head is present in about one-sixth of all cases. It is better to support the upper limb in a broad-arm sling and have good radiographs taken.

Reduction is performed in four ways: (i) the player lies prone on the couch with his injured arm hanging vertically for a few minutes, (ii) the stockinged foot of the doctor is placed in the player's axilla

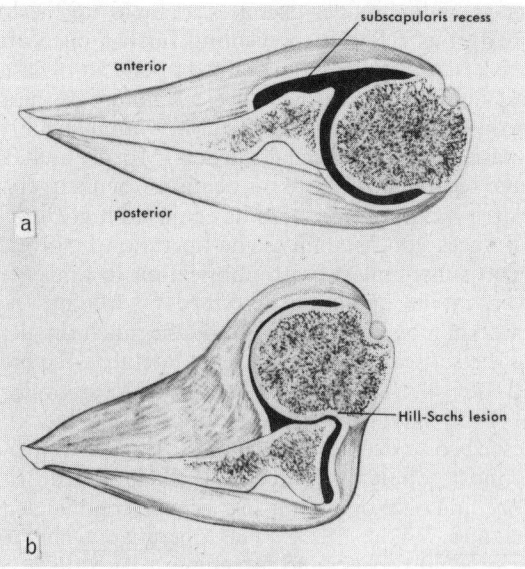

Fig. 47. Recurrent anterior dislocation of the shoulder. *a*, Laxity anteriorly, there is a large subscapularis recess with insertion of the anterior capsule far medially along the glenoid neck. *b*, This permits anterior subluxation and dislocation of the humeral head and the creation of a compression fracture in the posterolateral aspect of the head by the rim of the glenoid during anterior dislocation.

and the arm is gently pulled while foot pressure levers the humeral head into the glenoid cavity (Hippocratic method), (iii) Kocher's method, when the doctor pulls on the flexed elbow while the upper arm is abducted 15° and eased into full external rotation. The elbow is then carried forward and medially across the chest and when adduction is complete the arm is internally rotated, (iv) the elevation method which commences with the player lying on the table and the arm is gently elevated in forward flexion to the overhead position.

After reduction, shoulder movements are encouraged in a sling for 2–3 weeks and then formal abduction exercises begin. The common complications are an associated fracture (*Fig.* 46) (especially of the humeral head, tuberosity or surgical neck) tearing of the supraspinatus tendon, axillary nerve damage, brachial plexus injury and biceps tendon rupture.

RECURRENT DISLOCATION OF THE SHOULDER
Primary dislocation may have associated damage to the capsule or labrum at the glenoid rim (the Bankart lesion). There may also be a defect in the posterolateral aspect of the humeral head—the Hill–Sachs lesion (*Fig.* 47). Both factors militate against stability. Conservative treatment with shoulder exercises to build up the local muscle power is usually ineffective in preventing further dislocations. However, surgery is also unsuccessful in about 11 per cent of cases (Roberts, 1963; Morrey and Janes, 1976). Surgical failure is more frequent when there is a history of bilateral dislocation, a family history of dislocation, or the patient is in the teenage group (Morrey and Janes, 1976).

If there have been two or more dislocations then surgery is advised. The Putti–Platt procedure (*Fig.* 48*b*) has enjoyed a great deal of popularity and produces good stability. The operation involves incision of the capsule and subscapularis with imbrication to limit external rotation. However, in the operation described by Magnuson and Stack (1943) this external movement is limited by the much simpler procedure of advancing the subscapularis attachment lateral to the biceps tendon in its groove (*Fig.* 48*d*) although the overall results may not be as good as the Putti–Platt procedure. Various bone-block procedures have been described to deepen the glenoid fossa and to provide a bony buttress. The most popular and effective is the modified Bristow procedure (*Fig.* 48*a*) and this operation has been recommended in sportsmen (Collins and Wilde, 1973). The operative technique involves dividing the coracoid process and attaching it with the accompanying tendons to the anterior aspect of the glenoid fossa, just below its midpoint. It is necessary to incise the subscapularis and capsule to allow the passage of the bone and tendons to the fossa. Only skin and subcutaneous tissues are repaired once the coracoid has been screwed to the glenoid margin. The arm is immobilized for 4–6 weeks and then gentle antigravity exercises begin; at 8 weeks resisted exercises are commenced. Approximately 4 months elapse from surgery to sport, especially throwing events.

This operation accomplishes several things—it produces a bone block, a musculotendinous sling is introduced when the arm is externally rotated and abducted, and the lower half of the subscapularis is held low to reinforce the weaker antero-inferior area of the capsule.

In the Bankart repair (often combined with the Putti–Platt) the anterior edge of the glenoid fossa is roughed and small drill holes made (*Fig.* 48c). Through these holes the labrum and capsule are re-attached by sutures. After the combined procedure the arm is held by the side for 4–6 weeks and mobilization exercises begun.

The limitation of external rotation that results after a Putti–Platt and Bankart procedure is said to be greater than after a modified Bristow repair (Collins and Wilde, 1973). However, Lombardo et al. (1976) found that athletic individuals with involvement of the dominant shoulder were not capable of returning to high performance levels of overhead sports activity (particularly throwing) after the Bristow procedure, despite the fact that external rotation was limited by only 11°. A lack of power, velocity, strength and the necessary 'whipping' action at the extremes of external rotation were common complaints by competitive as well as recreational athletes—thus throwing a baseball, football or water polo ball was limited. Additionally they had problems with reaching (as in basketball or playing the positions of receiver and defensive back in American football, spiking in volleyball or serving in tennis, and in some cases swimming the backstroke).

POSTERIOR DISLOCATIONS OF THE SHOULDER
This injury is caused by a forced internal rotation of the abducted arm or by a blow on the shoulder in boxing. The clinical diagnosis is quite easy if the condition is considered, yet it is often missed for the anteroposterior radiograph looks relatively normal. However, axillary views reveal the dislocation. To achieve reduction the arm is pulled and rotated externally while the head of the humerus is pushed forwards. A sling is worn for 3 weeks.

SUBLUXATION OF THE SHOULDER
Blazina (1966) has stressed the importance of this condition in an athlete who has sustained an injury when there was a feeling that something had slipped out of joint. Radiographs are normal but the player is apprehensive when the arm is abducted and externally rotated. A generalized ache, localizing posteriorly, may be a feature and the shoulder may feel lax. Arthrography is often helpful in demonstrating

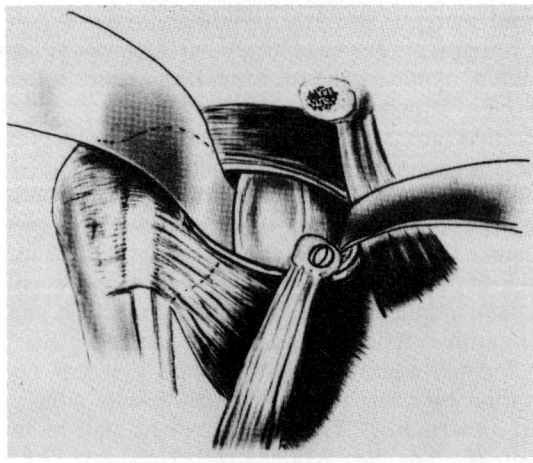

a

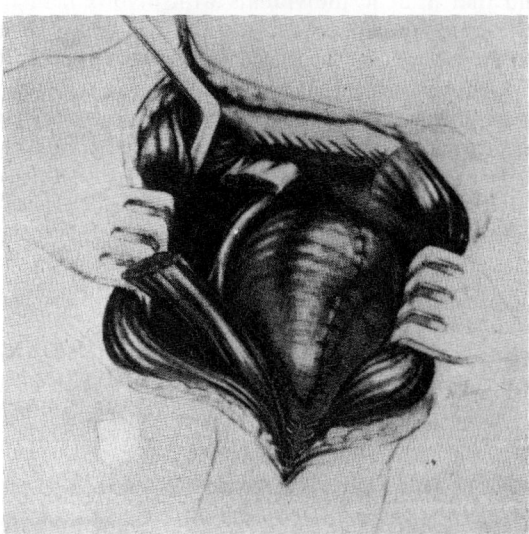

b

Fig. 48. Operations for recurrent dislocation of the shoulder. *a*, Bristow procedure. The coracoid process is attached to the anterior rim of the glenoid (Collins and Wilde, 1973). *b*, Putti–Platt procedure. The subscapularis tendon has been divided and the capsule incised. Sutures have been placed in the lateral part of subscapularis and in the soft structures along the anterior rim of the glenoid. These have been tied with the shoulder in internal rotation. Then the medial part of the subscapularis has been sutured to the rotator cuff at the greater tuberosity (Osmond-Clarke, 1948). *c*, Bankart procedure. Drill holes are made through the rim of the glenoid and the free incised lateral margin of the capsule and the detached labrum are sutured to the rim (Cave and Rowe, 1947). *d*, Magnuson procedure. The subscapularis insertion is transferred distally and laterally and stapled (or sutured) into a trough of raw bone. The new insertion is lateral to the biceps tendon (Rothman et al., 1975).

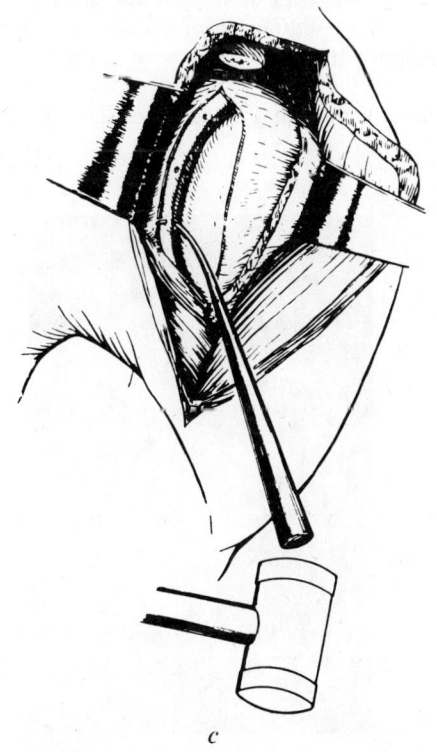

c

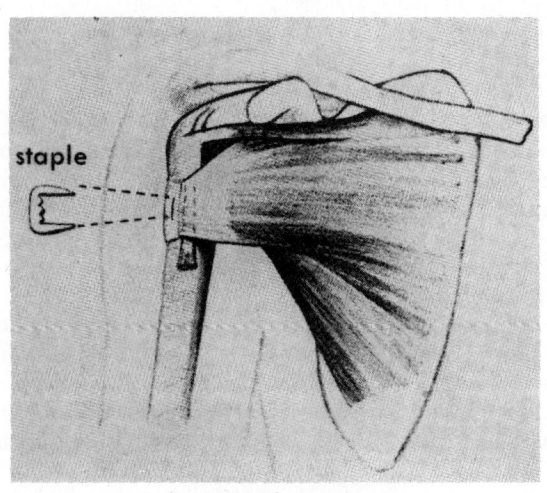

d

an enlarged pouch and tears of the rotator cuff (*Fig.* 49). Sometimes a Hill–Sachs lesion or a flattening of the anterior glenoid margin are seen on radiography. If subluxation becomes a problem due to pain or a feeling of instability then it is treated as a recurrent dislocation. In the first instance it is best treated by a high-arm sling for 4 weeks and exercises.

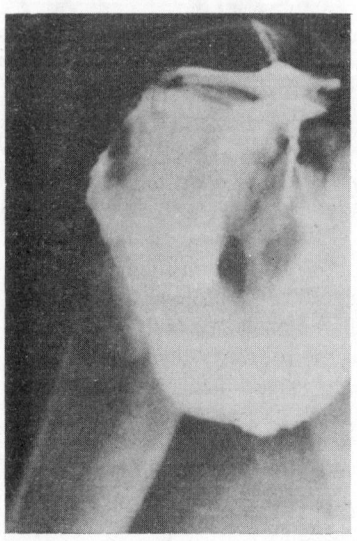

Fig. 49. An arthrogram of the shoulder showing anterior laxity in a case of chronic subluxation.

FRACTURES AND DISLOCATIONS AROUND THE ELBOW
The most serious fracture in a young athlete is the supracondylar fracture caused by a fall on the hand with a flexed elbow (*Fig.* 50*b*, *c*). Reduction is difficult in grossly displaced fractures with a large elbow haematoma. Undisplaced fractures need a simple plaster back-slab for 2–3 weeks. Displaced fractures can have the distal fragment either anterior or more commonly posterior to the humeral element. Reduction must disimpact the fracture and correct the lateral shift and medial rotation, but full flexion to lock the fragments may not be possible if the radial pulse becomes obliterated. Under these conditions Dunlop traction can be used. This consists of elevation of the forearm with an extended elbow using longitudinal traction and a pulley set just above bed height; countertraction is applied by weights suspended across the arm (Dunlop, 1939).

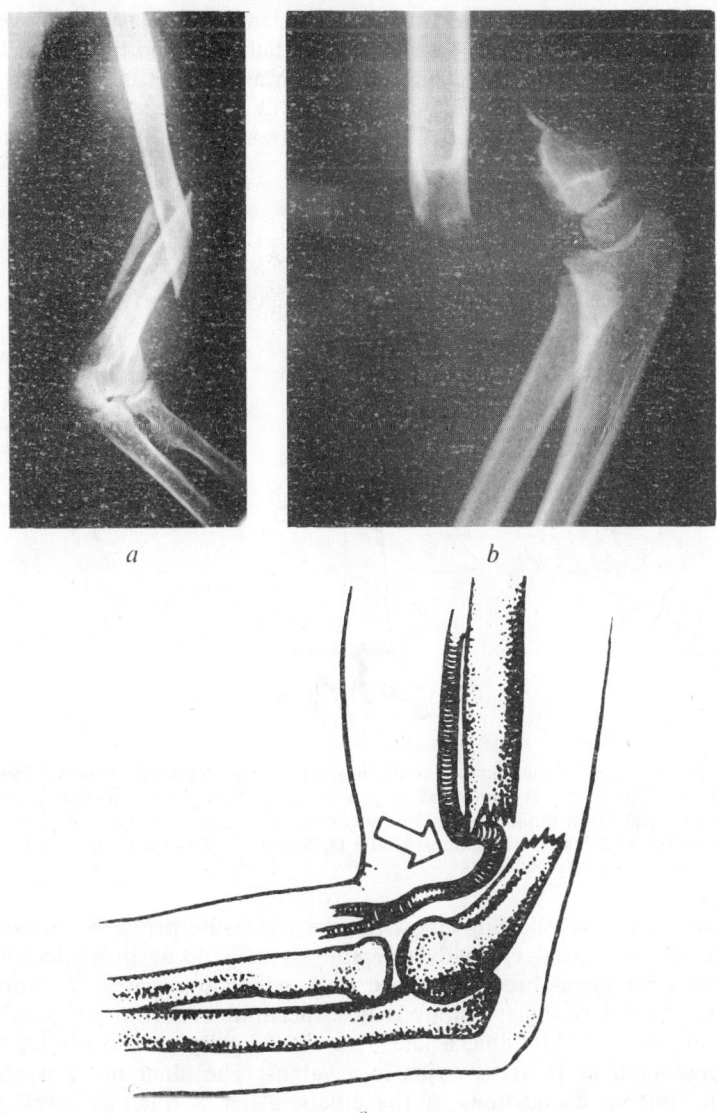

Fig. 50. Two serious injuries to the lower humerus: *a*, Comminuted spiral fracture Radial nerve injury and non-union are complications. Internal fixation may be required for realignment, to protect the damaged nerve from further movement, and to allow elbow mobility from an early stage. *b*, A posterior supracondylar fracture. *c*, Radiographs ignore the soft-tissue structures. Not only can the brachial artery be crushed, but the ulnar nerve and branches of the median and radial nerves can be damaged. A haemarthrosis develops in the joint, the capsule may be torn and the blood leaks into the soft tissues. The brachialis and triceps may be damaged.

A reduced supracondylar fracture is treated with a plaster back-slab and collar and cuff for 3-4 weeks. The radial pulse and finger circulation are watched throughout the reduction and for 48 hours after.

Most other long bone fractures are readily recognized (*Figs.* 51, 52) clinically and radiologically and their treatment follows standard orthopaedic practice.

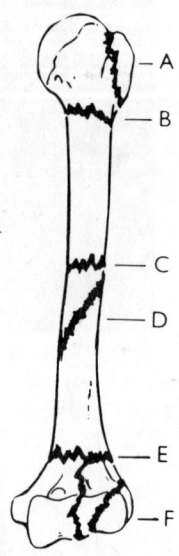

Fig. 51. Fractures of the humerus commonly found in athletes. Non-union is infrequent. Malalignment is controlled by gravity and the use of a plaster U-slab. Shoulder and elbow mobility should be encouraged from an early stage. A, Greater tuberosity; B, Neck; C, Transverse shaft: D, Spiral; E, T-shaped supracondylar; F, Lateral condyle.

However, the following elbow injuries can cause problems. Separation of the medial epicondylar epiphysis may occur in adolescents and the fragments become trapped in the elbow joint; while fractures of the lateral condylar epiphysis need accurate reduction to prevent non-union and malunion, a late ulnar nerve palsy can be the sequel to malunion as the elbow tilts into valgus. The ulnar nerve is also vulnerable in dislocations of the elbow. After a fractured neck of radius up to 15° of tilt is acceptable, more angulation requires open reduction.

Olecranon Fractures
The triceps may tear a small flake of bone from the tip of the olecranon in the javelin or other strenuous throwing events. This injury settles in

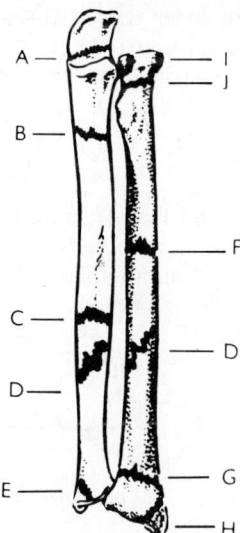

Fig. 52. Fractures of the radius and ulna commonly found in athletes. Malalignment often appears worse radiologically than clinically but rotation of the lower fragments can be missed leading to a diminished arc of supination/pronation. Displaced midshaft fractures with soft-tissue interposition may require internal fixation with compression plates. A, Olecranon; B, Shaft—ulna; C and D, Transverse or oblique fractures affecting both bones; E, Styloid—ulna; F, Shaft—radius; G, Colles; H, Styloid process—radius; I, Radial head; and J, neck of radius.

a broad arm sling for 2–3 weeks. However, with a fairly large olecranon fragment or in the presence of comminution the author favours tension band wiring which has the added advantage of early mobilization. For fractures half-way down the olecranon fossa the bone can be fixed with a large screw; it is removed under local anaesthesia 6–8 weeks later.

FRACTURES OF THE RADIUS AND ULNA

Special mention must be made of an isolated fracture of either the radius or ulna which is usually caused by a direct blow such as a kick on a goalkeeper's forearm in soccer. Because one bone is intact non-union is a possibility and internal fixation may be advisable. It is also worth pointing out that with an isolated fracture an associated dislocation may be missed and both radio-ulnar joints must be radiographed (i.e. a Monteggia fracture-dislocation when the radial head is dislocated and the ulna fractured; and a Galeazzi fracture-dislocation when the radial shaft is broken and the lower ulna dislocated).

The force which in an older person causes a Colles' fracture may, in a child, produce a fracture-separation of the lower radial epiphysis. Minor damage to the epiphysis may be passed off as a sprain; thus any tenderness over the lower radial epiphysis warrants a plaster for 3 weeks.

FRACTURED SCAPHOID
A fall on a dorsiflexed hand may fracture the scaphoid (*Fig.* 53) and pain in the anatomical snuffbox and a weak grip are found; on clinical suspicion alone the wrist is immobilized for 2–3 weeks in a scaphoid plaster even if radiographs are negative. Repeat films may show the fracture.

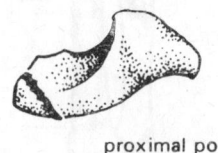
proximal pole

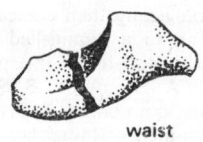
waist

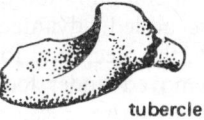
tubercle

Fig. 53. Fractures of the scaphoid.

In the presence of a fractured scaphoid the wrist is immobilized for up to 12 weeks but radiological union may take months to show. Persistent tenderness usually indicates non-union and the onset of avascular changes in the proximal pole. A bone graft can be carried out in the presence of non-union, or, in some instances, the avascular segment excised.

HAND FRACTURES
Such injuries are common in most sports and, for example, in hurling hand fracture may account for a quarter of all fractures. It is worth

recalling that fractures in this area almost always unite but that finger stiffness is a handicap both in sports and in everyday living; malunion is less disabling than stiffness. That is not to say that reduction should not be the aim, but attention should be directed at reducing swelling by hand elevation and promoting early movement by keeping splintage to a minimum.

With a simple phalangeal fracture the affected finger can be splinted to its neighbour, but if a plaster or metal splint is needed then the fingers are usually kept at 90° of flexion at the metacarpophalangeal joint, the remaining joints being held extended. Displaced fractures which cannot be reduced and held by closed methods require internal fixation with Kirschner wires or small plates and screws.

Bennett's Fracture
This is an intra-articular fracture-dislocation (*Fig.* 54*b*) which often requires internal fixation. This can be achieved by a small screw into the medial fragment across the fracture line. However, the small size of the fragment and the obliquity of the articular surface of the trapezium often require the fracture to be reduced by pulling on the thumb, abducting and extending. It is then transfixed by crossed Kirschner wires, which can pass into either the adjacent second metacarpal or the carpal bones. The wires are removed after 3 weeks. The alternative of closed reduction by the manoeuvre described above and a felt

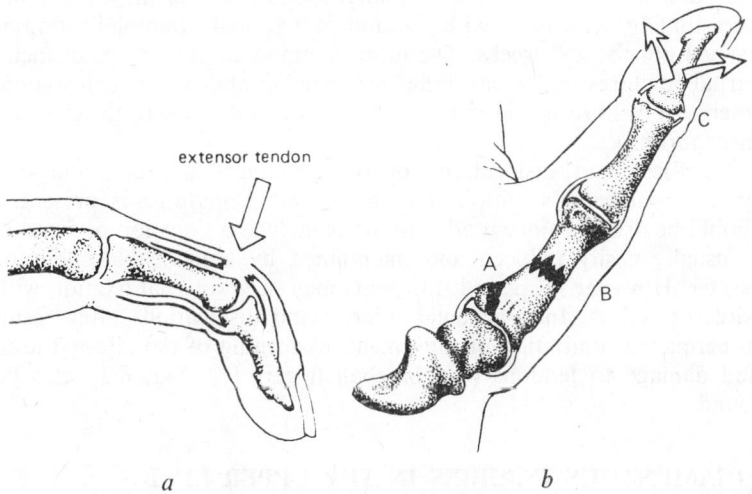

Fig. 54. Finger injuries. *a.* Mallet or baseball finger. *b,* Bennett's fracture (A); midshaft fracture (B) of the first metacarpal (boxer's thumb); rupture of the collateral ligaments (C).

pad over the fracture is effective in less than half the cases which the author has encountered: following all methods a plaster is worn for 4–6 weeks. Sport can begin after 6–8 weeks but in boxing and similar sports a 3–6 months' lay-off may be needed.

Metacarpal Fractures
Boxers frequently damage the first metacarpal base especially when training with heavy punch bags and poorly taped hands. Generally the fracture is transverse, a quarter of an inch distal to the carpometacarpal joint and reduction is performed by pulling on the abducted thumb and levering the metacarpal outwards against the operator's thumb, thus correcting the bowing. A firm crêpe bandage can be used but a plaster is preferred.

Spiral fractures and transverse fractures of the other metacarpal shafts with only slight displacement do not require reduction. However, when a punching injury has caused knuckle recession then the fracture is pulled to length and fixed with a plaster or by Kirschner wires; a small screw or plate can be employed but has to be removed before boxing can begin again.

Another common boxing fracture is of the fifth metacarpal neck. As in any metacarpal neck fracture slight displacement can be disregarded, but an ugly lump in the palm needs accurate reduction which is produced by direct thumb pressure in the palm. A thick pad of wool in the palm and a crêpe support holds the reduction in most cases but occasionally Kirschner wire fixation is required. Immobilization is carried out for 2–3 weeks. The most common complications of metacarpal fractures which can influence sporting ability are malrotation, interosseous fibrosis and intrinsic tightness and damage to the extensor mechanism.

Fractures and dislocations of the phalanges are common—the typical goalkeeper's injury. If a subungual haematoma is present it should be drained since it adds to the pain. The dislocation or fracture is usually easily reduced and maintained by a malleable splint or plaster. However, displaced fragments may need internal fixation with wires or screws. Intra-articular injuries and dislocations often result in permanent limitation of movement, thickening of the affected joint and damage to tendons (e.g. baseball finger, *Fig.* 54a) may also be found.

LIGAMENTOUS INJURIES IN THE UPPER LIMB
Rotator Cuff Tears
The attenuated insertions of the rotator cuff are usually torn while the fleshy parts remain intact. Degenerative changes are not usually

a factor in the injury process in athletes. Tears may be partial or complete.
There are four mechanisms for rotator cuff damage:
1. Throwing. The velocity of the whirling head of the humerus is applied to the anterior capsule, with subsequent labrum loosening, subluxation and rupture of the capsule and subscapularis.
2. A direct fall onto the shoulder may tear the capsule as well as causing a fracture of the humeral tuberosity. This displaced fragment can distort the normal overhanging arch leading to subacromial bursitis and interfering with shoulder mobility.
3. A vertical thrust through an extended limb can be transmitted to the capsular structures. Normally the arm is held in abduction and flexion during a fall and the forces are transmitted through the bony structure. When the arm is kept by the side the soft tissues suffer most; such an accident occurs in skiing because skiers tend to hold the poles close to the body.
4. Cuff injuries accompany shoulder dislocations.

DIAGNOSIS
When the supraspinatus tendon is damaged (*Fig.* 55) pain is felt radiating from the deltoid insertion and there is difficulty in initiating abduction of the arm. Passive abduction is also limited by pain. It may be difficult to distinguish between partial and complete tears at this stage. However, once the pain has been abolished by local anaesthesia, with partial tears the patient can abduct the limb. With complete tears active abduction is impossible and attempting it produces a characteristic shrug; but abduction is full once the arm has been passively lifted above 90° when the patient can maintain it by deltoid action (the abduction paradox). The treatment of supraspinatus injuries is by heat and exercises in partial tears but the early repair of complete tears is advisable.

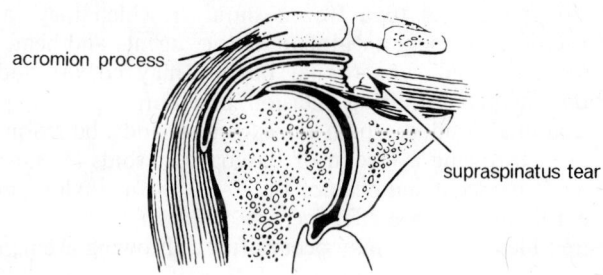

Fig. 55. Supraspinatus tear.

Tears of the anterior capsule may present with shoulder soreness in throwing events or after a fall and, on attempting to throw, a sharp pain and a feeling of instability are experienced. Unlike supraspinatus tears the player has a full range of circumduction including abduction. However, shoulder movements are weak and can be easily overcome by the examiner, gentle pressure stopping abduction. Clinical examination also reveals tenderness over the anterior capsule and anterior laxity of the humeral head can be elicited.

Plain radiographs do not help but an arthrogram will reveal the tear in the rotator cuff or anterior capsule.

TREATMENT

The rotator cuff tear is repaired using either an axillary approach or an anterosuperior approach. The former is comparatively bloodless, avoids damage to tendons and muscles and gives a neat scar. However, access may be limited and the anterosuperior incision is to be preferred in the presence of bulky muscles. The coraco-acromial ligament can be divided to allow full inspection and mobilization of the rotator cuff. All adhesions are divided and the torn surfaces trimmed; the edges are sutured with dexon. If the tuberosity of the humerus has been avulsed the small piece of bone is removed and the cuff is laid over the defect so that it lies flush with the bone and does not impinge on the arch during an overhead swing.

Bateman (1969) has described a repair of the anterior capsule and subscapularis using fascial strips darned across the defect; they are anchored in the scapula just anterior to the labrum and into the humerus just lateral to the insertion of the subscapularis. An abduction splint is worn for 3 weeks but gentle abduction exercises begin after 7 days with lowering of the splint.

Painful Shoulders

Capsulitis results from a sprain in which the degree of violence is not sufficient to provoke more than a transient subluxation. Sometimes the condition progresses to a frozen shoulder which may take 6–9 months to settle even using anti-inflammatory agents and heat. Supraspinatus tendinitis and subacromial bursitis may coexist and show ectopic bony masses requiring incision and curettage (Chapter 5). Bicipital tendinitis produces pain on extension and abduction of the shoulder as in throwing a javelin or baseball. Steroids (50 mg hydrocortisone in 2 per cent lignocaine; or 20–30 mg methylprednisolone in 2 per cent lignocaine) are effective.

A ruptured biceps tendon may occur after a throwing event; usually in a patient over 45 years of age. A sensation of snapping is felt in the arm and the bunched biceps muscle is obvious. The Hitchcock repair

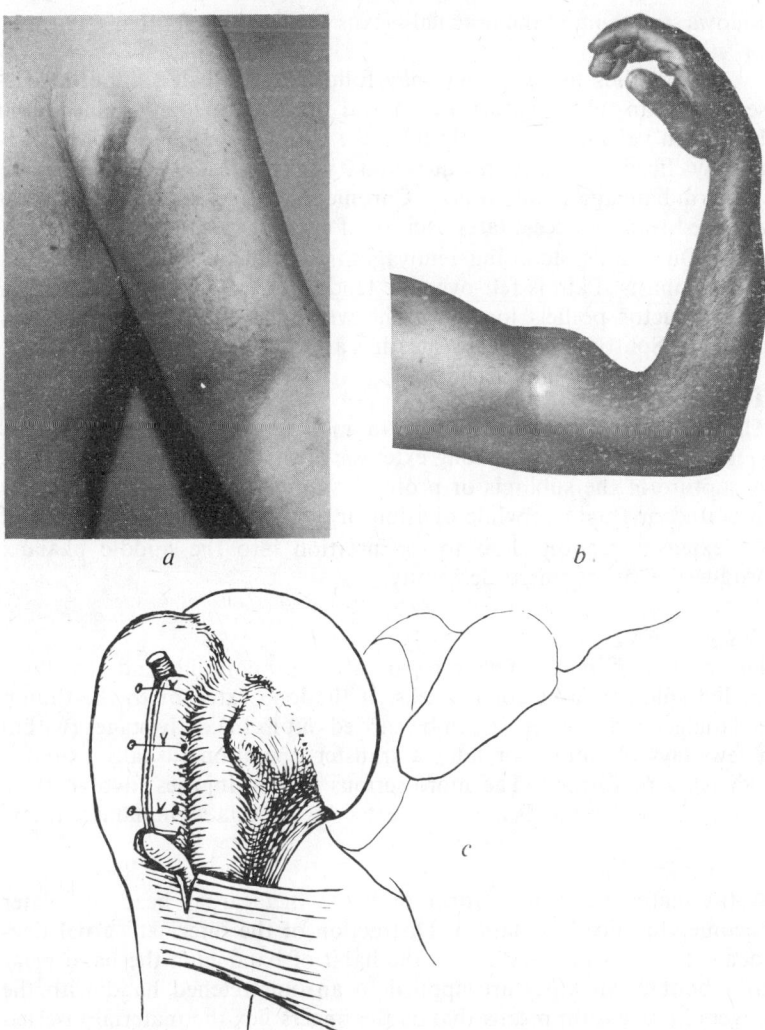

Fig. 56. *a,* Rupture of the biceps muscle in a rugby player. *b,* Rupture of the long head of biceps. *c,* Hitchcock method of anchoring the ruptured long head of biceps (Crenshaw and Kilgore, 1966).

is depicted in *Fig.* 56 but usually the tear occurs through a degenerative area in the long head and surgical repair may not be feasible; good results often follow simple shoulder exercises. Rupture of the lower tendon of biceps at the elbow is uncommon and treated by surgical repair (Boyd and Anderson, 1961). Bicipital pain and weakness follows stretching of the brachial plexus in American football ('burners' or 'stingers').

Loose bodies in the elbow may follow injury, osteochondritis dissecans or an inflammatory lesion and need removing. An olecranon bursa can be caused by a fall on to the elbow as in judo. Aspiration is usually effective in an acute injury and 2 weeks of rest of the injured area in a firm bandage should follow. Chronic thickening of the bursa due to repeated trauma necessitates excision if swelling becomes a problem.

De Quervain's stenosing tenovaginitis occurs in volleyball players and gymnasts. Pain is felt over the tendons of extensor pollicis brevis and abductor pollicis longus at the wrist and the thickened area is palpable. Splitting the fibrous sheath is a simple operation and effective.

Tendon Injuries in the Fingers

The commonest tendon injury is a mallet finger or baseball finger (*Fig.* 54a); sometimes the long extensor of the thumb can be involved. A rupture of the sublimis or profundus alone or together may follow a wound or fracture; while division or avulsion of the central slip of the extensor tendon close to its insertion into the middle phalanx produces a boutonnière deformity.

TREATMENT

The results of mallet finger repair are disappointing and usually a 'mallet splint' is used for 6 weeks. If the long extensor to the thumb is damaged a direct repair can be carried out in the early stages (within a few days of injury) or later a transfer operation (usually extensor indicis) is performed. The more serious tendon injuries involving the profundus and sublimis are best treated by a specialist in hand surgery.

Boxer's Knuckle

A traumatic bursa may form over the metacarpal head and later become chronically inflamed. Distraction of the intermetacarpal ligaments can also be painful and the habit of bandaging the hand prior to a bout when tapes are applied to an outstretched hand with the fingers in extension means that as the fingers flex the material inserted between them causes distraction of these ligaments. The treatment of both these conditions is by analgesics and correct bandaging (Sperryn, 1973).

Participants in racket games such as squash and badminton may injure their pisotriquetral joint, resulting in pain on the inner side of the hand and wrist. Repeated backward and forward twisting movements of the wrist aggravate the pain. Excision of the pisiform has been advocated if rest and infiltration with a local anaesthetic are not effective.

Chapter 11

Injuries to the head and face

Any minor head injury needs special consideration to exclude serious neurological complications. Glancing or tangential blows produce this injury in soccer and rugby while in American football the 'head-on' tackle can cause both head and cervical spine trauma. Only in boxing is violence aimed at producing a period of concussion but in many sports a missile-type injury can be produced by a hard ball, flying racket or contact with an opponent's boot or the ground.

BRAIN INJURY
In any head injury it is the brain damage that matters most. It is well recognized that a fatal brain injury may occur without blemish to the scalp or a skull fracture. The simplest form of brain injury is concussion, the essential feature of this condition being its reversibility, with complete recovery occurring within a few seconds or minutes. Electroencephalogram studies have confirmed that changes in rhythm do not persist for more than 4 minutes (Blonstein, 1960). In more severe cases there may be brain laceration or contusion particularly if the skull is fractured. Secondary complicating factors such as haemorrhage, cerebral oedema and late infection may ensue. Since cerebral oedema is aggravated by a fall in oxygen level a good airway must always be preserved in unconscious players.

Diagnosis
There is usually a loss of consciousness; confusion, irritability, headache, nausea, vomiting, photophobia and double vision are often present. Serious signs are increasing confusion, dilated or irregular

pupils, rapid and feeble pulse, rapid respiration, and weakness and sensory disturbances in the limbs including ataxia.

Associated Conditions
1. Scalp wounds.
2. Skull fracture.
3. Traumatic intracranial haemorrhage.
4. Neck or spinal injury.
5. Facial injury.

SCALP WOUNDS
These bleed freely and may require adrenaline in the local anaesthetic; all layers of the scalp split as one and are sutured accordingly. The base of the wound should be examined for a fracture.

SKULL FRACTURE
Classified as simple or compound; linear, comminuted or depressed (*Fig.* 57). Classically a boggy swelling is found over the fracture. Blows to the nasal or frontal region may injure the delicate cribriform plate with resulting rhinorrhoea. A black eye appearing some hours later with little or no damage to the skin around the eye and with a flame-shaped subconjunctival haemorrhage indicates a fractured anterior fossa. Blood in the ear which does not clot due to admixture with cerebrospinal fluid indicates a middle or posterior fossa fracture. The latter fracture may also produce a boggy swelling at the nape of the neck or behind the mastoid process.

TRAUMATIC INTRACRANIAL HAEMORRHAGE
This may be: (*a*) subcortical, (*b*) subdural, (*c*) extradural.

Subcortical bleeding occurs on or within the soft brain substance and may be associated with a brain laceration. *Subdural bleeding* is caused by venous injury (*Fig.* 57*c*) with associated pulping of the brain tissue. *Extradural bleeding* results from an injury to the meningeal vessels, the usual cause being a laterally directed blow, often trivial, such as occurs from a golf or cricket ball, which strikes the thin temporal plate. The classic extradural haemorrhage syndrome (*Fig.* 57*d*) has a brief period of unconsciousness followed by a lucid interval when the player may apparently act normally; later becoming confused and then unconscious as the bleeding progresses.

Treatment of a Head Injury
After mild concussion the player should abandon the match and be taken for a skull radiograph. It is very difficult, on many occasions, to get the player to agree to both these requests especially if there has been only a very brief period of unconsciousness. Nevertheless

the club doctor must take a firm stand, also insisting that the player rests for 24 hours after the injury. Although most sportsmen are anxious to start training the next day a period of 3–5 days of rest is advisable, while in some contact sports (e.g. rugby, soccer, American football) a much longer period of 1–3 weeks has been advocated.

Boxers are a special problem. The majority of boxers who have been knocked out can get up at the end of the count, indeed most attempt to do so between 5 and 8. Generally they can walk to the corner where they quickly recover. Usually there is no retrograde amnesia, headache or vomiting and neurological examination is nearly always negative. However, boxers who have been concussed should not fight again for 2–3 months.

With a serious head injury the player is transferred to a neurosurgical unit. Traumatic epilepsy may complicate 5 per cent of all major closed injuries. After repeated head injuries (e.g. boxing, steeplechase riding) the participant should be warned of the long-term dangers and advised to give up the sport.

Headaches, nausea, dizziness and poor concentration (often called the minor head injury syndrome) may follow brief periods of unconsciousness and may persist for several weeks. An immediate 24 hours of bed rest, preferably in hospital, seems to reduce the frequency of this slight but troublesome complication. The presence of papilloedema and other neurological signs occurring weeks after a head injury requires investigation to exclude chronic subdural haematoma.

Prevention of Head Injuries
Protective headgear such as crash helmets in motor cycle events and motor racing and the lighter hard skull caps in cycling, horse-riding and skiing will protect against head injuries. Headgear should also be worn during training in boxing, and as an additional safeguard during a bout the ring floor should be covered by felt or sorbo-rubber 15 mm thick. The latter measure has reduced both the severity and frequency of injury since it was introduced to lessen the impact on the falling boxer. Gum shields also soften the blows to the jaws which are, in turn, transmitted to the skull.

Traumatic encephalopathy, commonly called 'punch drunkenness', has declined over the past 50 years. The typical clinical features are probably due to diffuse brain cell damage with petechial haemorrhages in and around the brain stem. The term 'punch drunk' accurately and graphically describes the boxer who is unsteady on his feet, euphoric, quarrelsome, with slurred speech and intellectual impairment. The referee's intervention to stop bouts when one boxer is definitely outclassed or is dazed, the compulsory count to 8 when one

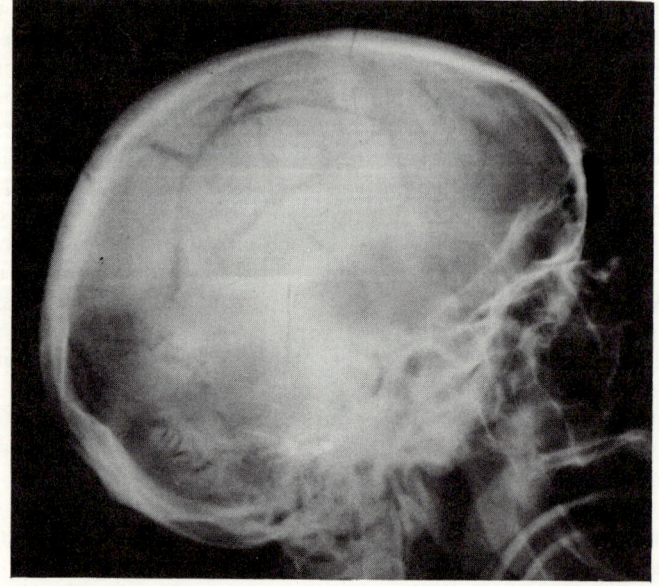

a

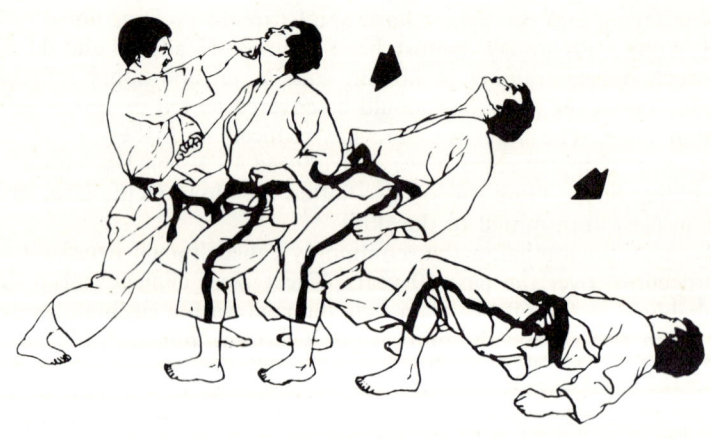

b

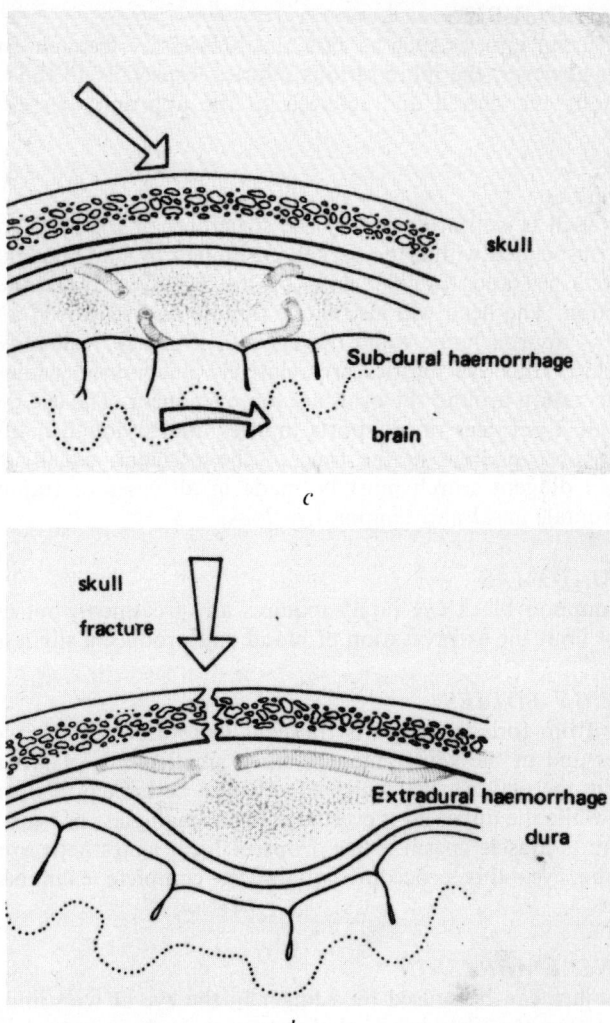

Fig. 57. *a*, Linear fractures of the skull. *b*, Serious head and neck injuries can occur after a competitor falls heavily against a hard surface (McLatchie, 1979). *c*, Subdural haematoma. *d*, Extradural haematoma.

boxer is knocked down and the continuation of the count at the end of a round when the boxer is still down, the limitation of amateur contests to three rounds, and the recommendation that amateur boxers should retire at 25 years—all these measures have gone a long way to eliminating this syndrome.

FACIAL INJURIES
Minor facial injuries such as cuts and bruises are frequent in contact sports; however, the more serious injuries, especially to the eye, must be readily recognized and referred to the appropriate specialist for advice.

Eye Injuries
The eyeball is well protected by the structures of the hard bony orbit and is suspended within the socket, cushioned by fat. The blink reflex, the eyelashes and forcible close of the eyelids all provide further protection. The head will also move rapidly and reflexly if a speeding object is approaching; while the eyeball, if struck, will move within the orbit. Thus eye injuries are relatively uncommon while bruising and laceration around the orbit are more frequent. The eye is involved in about 2 per cent of all sports injuries and although many serious injuries are apparent at the time of the accident, usually by visual upset, a diligent search must be made in all cases of trauma to the eye, frontal, nasal and temporal regions.

HAEMATOMAS
The common black eye rarely requires any treatment, but cold compresses limit the extravasation of blood and produce a slight analgesia.

FOREIGN BODIES
Injury from foreign bodies is frequent in football matches on dusty pitches and in the winter months when small pieces of grit and mud lodge in the player's eye, which then has to be bathed in warm, sterile saline while the upper lid is everted using a small glass rod as a fulcrum. If there is muscle spasm a few drops of local anaesthetic are instilled into the eye—this procedure will allow complete examination and lavage.

CORNEAL ABRASION
This injury can be caused by a finger in the eye at wrestling or water polo. Often the player feels that a foreign body is lodged in the eye but fluorescein dye will outline the abrasion. Symptoms settle in 2 days; at the most the immediate treatment consists of cleaning the eye with a mild antibiotic solution and a sterile eye-pad is worn.

SUBCONJUNCTIVAL HAEMORRHAGE
No treatment is needed and resolution occurs in 7–10 days. However, the eye must be carefully examined for other injuries such as vitreous haemorrhage and retinal detachment.

ANTERIOR CHAMBER HAEMORRHAGE
This can be caused by a ball or stick, or a clash of heads at soccer. Blood is seen in the anterior chamber obscuring the pupil and iris; later, a fluid level is formed. An eye pad is applied as a first aid measure and urgent ophthalmic advice sought. The haemorrhage usually absorbs in 7 days.

OTHER SERIOUS EYE INJURIES
A penetrating injury can occur from a flying missile or broken racket. There is immediate loss of vision and prolapse of the iris.

Repeated or severe trauma to the orbit and temporal region can cause choroid or vitreous injuries, lens prolapse, retinal oedema and retinal detachment. The latter serious condition frequently begins with a small retinal break (dialysis) which appears in the periphery (usually temporal). However, retinal detachment may not occur for many weeks and it is important to diagnose the dialysis before this happens. After ophthalmic surgery the sportsman is usually advised to give up contact sports, especially boxing, wrestling and judo. It goes without saying that an exponent of these sports who complains of persistent visual problems should be suspected of a retinal injury.

PREVENTION OF EYE INJURIES
All eye injuries must be taken seriously from the outset until proved relatively innocent by ophthalmic examination. Every sportsman must have good vision and defects should be treated by glasses or contact lenses. In sports such as hockey, cricket, tennis and athletics the frames should be strong and have splinterproof lenses. Soft contact lenses are especially suitable in sporting events. Short-sighted people should be discouraged from boxing because of the danger of retinal detachment and a similar caution applies to front-row forwards in rugby, as well as to wrestling, American football and judo exponents. Skiers, yachtsmen and water-skiers should wear filtering spectacles or goggles against scattered ultraviolet light. In competitive swimming, swimmers may cover several thousand metres per week during training. Sore eyes are produced because the water is not isotonic with lacrimal fluid; thus goggles with well-padded rims and non-splinter glass should be used.

Ear
Haematomas of the auricle ('cauliflower ear') are caused by shearing forces; the smaller peripheral haematoma is due to small-vessel bleeding but the larger haematomas are produced by rupture of the auricular artery or vein and the whole ear may be involved. All haematomas require incision and drainage since the extravasation of blood lifts

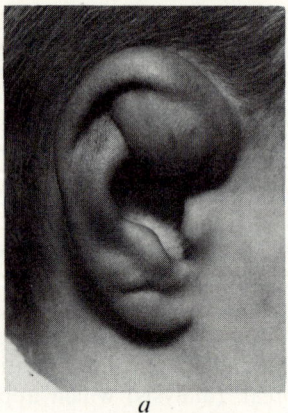
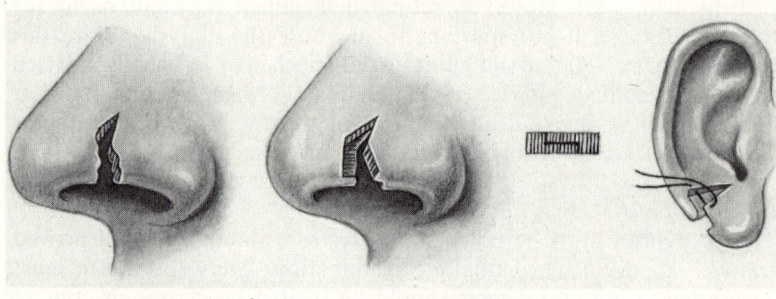

Fig. 58. *a*, Haematoma of the pinna with perichondritis. (From *Hamilton Bailey's Demonstrations of Physical Signs in Clinical Surgery*.) *b*, Halving and stepping applied to a laceration of the nose. *c*, Similar procedure with an ear laceration (From *Hamilton Bailey's Emergency Surgery*.)

the perichondrium off the cartilage which becomes necrotic and replaced by fibrous tissue.

After incision and drainage a pressure dressing is applied and play can be resumed after 2 weeks. Thereafter a sweat band with padding should be worn.

Old haematomas require evacuation of the fluid contents and heal by granulation tissue.

Nose

Fractures (*Fig.* 59) require either immediate reduction or delayed reduction for 4 days or so until the swelling has subsided. Displaced cartilages and nasal septum are similarly treated, but these injuries can be specially troublesome if they cause unilateral nasal obstruction. Sometimes a submucous haematoma can cause similar symptoms and needs incision under local anaesthesia. Cosmetic surgery for nasal deformity is best delayed until the end of a playing career in contact sports.

Epistaxis is common in boxing and many other sports and can be combated by gently pinching the nose and applying pressure with a cold sponge. Nasal packing with an adrenaline solution may be required. After a broken nose, unless there was marked comminution,

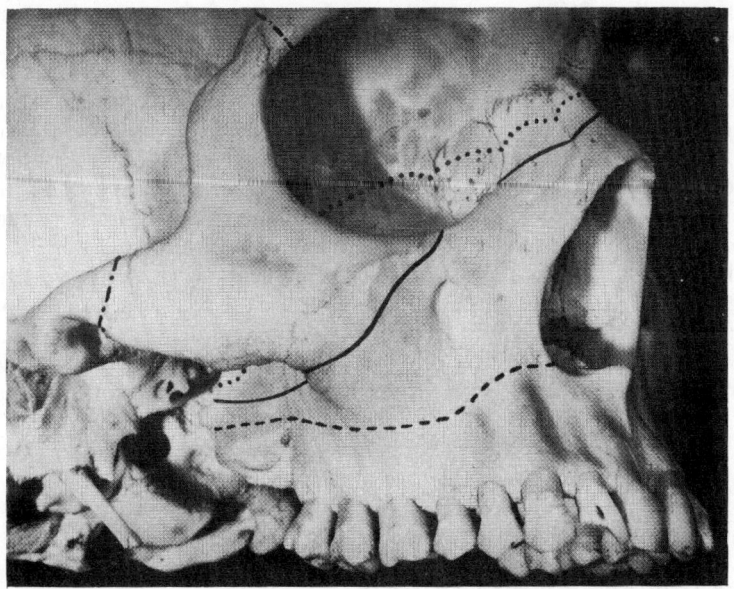

Fig. 59. Fractures in the middle and lower thirds of the face. Le Fort 1 (broken line); Le Fort 2 (solid line); Le Fort 3 (dotted line) (Killey, 1968).

contact sport can be resumed within 2–3 weeks although in boxing a 2–3 months' lay-off may be necessary.

Facial Fractures

These are complex injuries affecting, in the main, the middle third and lower third (mandible). Killey (1968) has divided middle third fractures into six subgroups (nasal complex; zygomatic complex; Le Fort 1 or low level fracture; Le Fort 2, the pyramidal fracture; Le Fort 3, the high level fracture; and dento-alveolar fractures) (*Fig.* 59).

MIDDLE THIRD FRACTURES

Maxillofacial injuries (*Fig.* 59) are usually easy to recognize by the obvious bony deformity, swelling and ecchymosis, and fracture should always be suspected if the teeth do not occlude properly.

The care of middle third injuries requires expert surgical advice but certain features are pertinent in sports medicine. Zygomatic fractures (*Fig.* 59) occur during a clash of heads at soccer. The face is slightly flattened but this may be masked by oedema. Mandibular movements may be impeded and double vision and anaesthesia in the distribution of the infraorbital nerve are commonly found. Unilateral epistaxis is also a salient feature, indeed these fractures are often missed because radiographs are relied upon rather than physical signs. Reduction is required to cure diplopia, free mandibular movements and restore the normal anatomy. However, slightly displaced fractures causing no symptoms do not warrant surgery.

An associated blow-out fracture of the orbital floor is a serious complication. This injury is caused by a sudden rise in intraorbital pressure as a hard ball strikes the rim of the orbit. There is circumorbital ecchymosis, subconjunctival haemorrhage and epistaxis, while clouding of the maxillary sinus may be evident on radiography. Diplopia, enophthalmos and limitation of eye movements are serious signs and require expert advice. This injury should always be suspected in contact sports when the player receives an accidental kick in the orbital region; the author has seen it on occasions in goalkeepers diving for a low ball.

The complex Le Fort fractures have been reviewed by Killey (1968) and generally require reduction and splintage with dental wires or extraoral fixation devices. Depending on the severity of the injury the athlete may not be able to compete for 3–6 months.

FRACTURES OF THE MANDIBLE

Rowe and Killey (1968) reported that 27 per cent of all mandibular fractures were caused by fighting. The diagnosis is obvious as there is pain, swelling, ecchymosis and bleeding from the mouth. The mandible is readily palpable from within the mouth (*Fig.* 59).

Fractures in the ramus area (condylar region, coronoid process, and ramus fractures) are usually treated by early movement. Fractures in the body area (fracture of the angle, mid-body fracture, fractures lateral to the midline in the incisor area and alveolar fractures) often require reduction and immobilization, the type of splintage employed depending upon the number and distribution of the teeth present. Fractures take 6–8 weeks to unite and oral hygiene is important to prevent infection.

Dislocation of the mandible is usually unilateral but may be bilateral. It can occur with a blow on the partially open mouth. Reduction is carried out by pressing the padded thumbs on the lower molar teeth

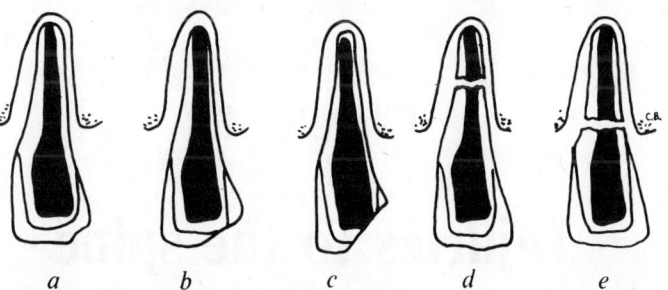

Fig. 60. Injuries to the teeth. *a*, The enamel is broken. *b*, The dentine is exposed. *c*, The nerve root is exposed. *d*, A fracture close to the root apex. *e*, A fracture at gum level. (The outcome in *d* is more favourable than in *e*.)

and rotating the chin forwards and inwards; general anaesthesia may be needed. A support is worn for 1-3 weeks.

Injuries to the teeth
Fig. 60 shows the types of teeth injuries. If the dentine or the nerve are exposed immediate treatment is needed to prevent tooth death and a dental abscess. A fracture close to the root requires crowning. When a tooth is knocked out it should be retrieved, washed in sterile saline (if possible) and reinserted at once. The tooth is held in the socket using gauze and gentle pressure expels the blood and tissue fluids. Once implanted, the tooth is kept in position by dental pressure until advice is available. It is important that the root area is not scrubbed or wiped vigorously.

A gum shield will prevent dental injuries. The stock gum shield may not be adapted to individual mouths and a shield of latex has been advocated in rugby and related sports (McGlashan, 1976). However, gum shields carry the risk of choking when a player has been concussed by a blow in the face.

Chapter 12

Injuries to the spine

Ligamentous sprains and pulled muscle fibres are common spinal problems but rarely inconvenience the athlete for more than a week or so. However, backache due to a prolapse of an intervertebral disc, a bony abnormality or osteoarthrosis of the facet joints is more refractory to treatment and is thus responsible for longer periods of incapacity than the simple sprains and contusions. Even direct kicks and blows to the spine rarely damage the vertebral bodies, discs and appendages. More troublesome is the collision at speed, as for example in American football or in rugby, which added to the normal momentum produces a twisting force. This force causes shearing of the posterior ligamentous complex and possible dislocation or fracture-dislocation of the facet joints and intervertebral disc damage.

SPRAINS
These are common in all athletic pursuits, especially weight-lifting, hammer and javelin throwing. Young tennis players with a poor serve often develop backstrain, as do 'one-sided' oarsmen. The treatment is rest and analgesics and although this condition usually remits very quickly, faulty techniques must be corrected to prevent recurrence.

FRACTURES AND DISLOCATIONS OF THE SPINE
On clinical and radiological grounds these injuries can be divided into stable and unstable (*Fig.* 61); the latter being associated with serious disruptive bony or ligamentous instability and thus more liable to involve the spinal cord or peripheral nerves. In rugby about 3 per cent of injuries involve the cervical spine but paraplegia and death are uncommon. In American football 12 fatalities occur annually from cervical spine injuries and in an analysis of 225 serious injuries

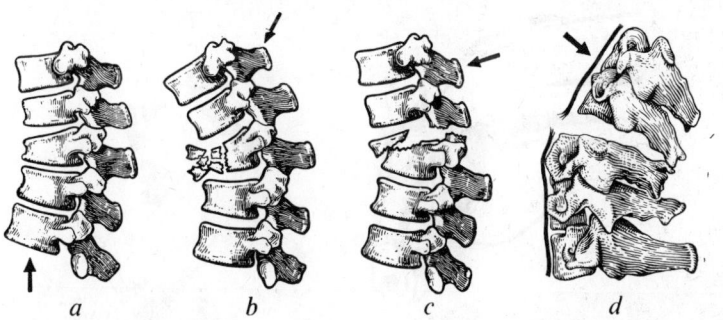

Fig. 61. *a*, Crush fracture. *b*, Comminuted fracture. *c*, Fracture-dislocation. *d*, Hyperextension rupture of the anterior longitudinal ligament. (*c* and *d* are unstable because of associated ligamentous injuries.) (From *Hamilton Bailey's Emergency Surgery*.)

and deaths in this sport almost three-quarters were due to cervical spine dislocations (Kyle, 1976).

Stable Fractures
These involve the spinous processes, transverse processes and laminae; they also include the compression fracture of the vertebral body. Most can be treated on an outpatient basis using analgesics, lumbar supports or plaster jackets or a collar but during the acute phase a few days of bed rest may be required; it is rarely needed for more than 1–2 weeks. Sport can begin with light mobilization exercises at 3–4 weeks and full activity 2 weeks later. Some discomfort may persist for several weeks but gradually subsides.

Unstable Fractures
These are common in areas of maximum mobility (C5 to C7; and in the thoracolumbar region, T12 to L2) especially after riding accidents (*Fig.* 62). In all unstable fractures there is soft-tissue disruption of the posterior spinal ligaments, sometimes with separation through a disc or a pedicle fracture. This soft-tissue injury is a key factor in the treatment of unstable fractures and must never be forgotten.

CERVICAL SPINE INJURIES
Compression, hyperextension and a combination of flexion and rotation are the movements which cause these injuries.

Compression injuries occur in diving into shallow water, trampoline exercises, high jumping and pole vaulting. Hyperextension injuries occur in American football with a tackle from behind or when the chin is in collision with a knee or the ground. However, in American football the players are taught how to use their heads and necks in

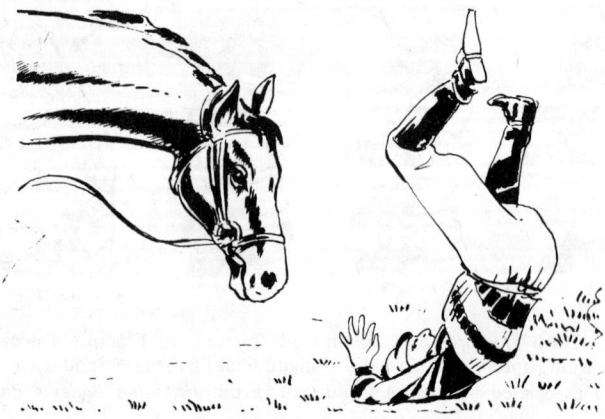

Fig. 62. Typical horse-riding injury pattern to head, cervical spine, thoracolumbar junction and shoulder. Sometimes the horse may roll over the jockey's pelvis or lower limb.

tackling and their heads and shoulders are heavily protected in contradistinction to rugby players. Flexion injuries are caused in rugby with collapse of the scrum, in the mêlée of the line-out and in head-on tackles. Wrestling also has a proportion of lateral rotational injuries to the neck.

Diagnosis
All cervical injuries produce local pain sometimes with radiation to the upper limbs, while weakness may be present in both the arms and legs after cord damage. Since clinical examination of the neck may only reveal muscle spasm good radiographs are essential and should include C7 which is often missed on the lateral film, an open-mouth view of the odontoid peg and, if necessary, oblique views and flexion/extension films. Commonly a subluxation or a unilateral dislocation is missed unless these investigations are thoroughly performed; and a tomogram is useful if a unilateral dislocation is suspected. The author has seen players with the latter injury continuing to undertake light training exercises despite unremitting neck ache because the radiological examination was not thorough enough.

Treatment
Stable fractures are treated with a removable polythene collar or plaster collar for 6–8 weeks.

Unstable fractures and dislocations need immobilization and reduction. This can be accomplished by Crutchfield's tongs and after a period of several days, when the facets have been reduced and the haematoma has subsided, a bone grafting operation is carried out since the posterior spinal ligaments heal poorly and thus do not provide long term stability. The grafted area is protected by traction for 2–3 weeks and a collar (usually made of plaster initially) is employed for a further 9–10 weeks. In the same way a Minerva plaster can be used for 6–12 weeks in odontoid fractures which have been reduced by skull traction. When carrying out a radiological assessment of the dens it is wise to seek expert advice since congenital abnormalities may be confused with fracture lines and vice versa. The un-united odontoid causes special problems due to neck ache and instability; usually an occipitocervical fusion (or C1 to C2 fusion) is performed.

Although plaster collars have been used after the reduction of a cervical spine dislocation, Durbin (1957) showed that even after 6 months of such immobilization redisplacement can occur; hence the need for surgical intervention and grafting.

THORACIC, LUMBAR AND THORACOLUMBAR INJURIES

Forced flexion, shearing forces and hyperextension tend to cause these injuries. Forced flexion is common after falls at speed (e.g. motor cycle and horse-riding accidents) but the posterior ligaments remain intact. However, with shearing forces, such as occur when the body is thrown and twisted at the same time, a slice of bone may be sheared off the top of one vertebra and the posterior facets fractured. This is a very unstable fracture because of the extensive disruption of soft tissues which causes a boggy swelling within an hour or so but a palpable gap between the spinous processes is found in the lumbar fascia at once. Hyperextension injuries occur with a tackle from behind or may occur with a collision at speed. The principal fracture is of the laminae.

Diagnosis

Pain is experienced in the affected areas and may radiate to the abdominal or chest wall (thus mimicking visceral injury) and to the legs. Anteroposterior and lateral radiographs should be taken and, if there is any doubt, two laterals are required, one centred over the vertebral bodies, the other over the spinous processes.

Treatment

The player is removed without altering his position (so he should not be moved until there are enough competent helpers) with gentle traction applied to the head and legs and the spine firmly supported on a

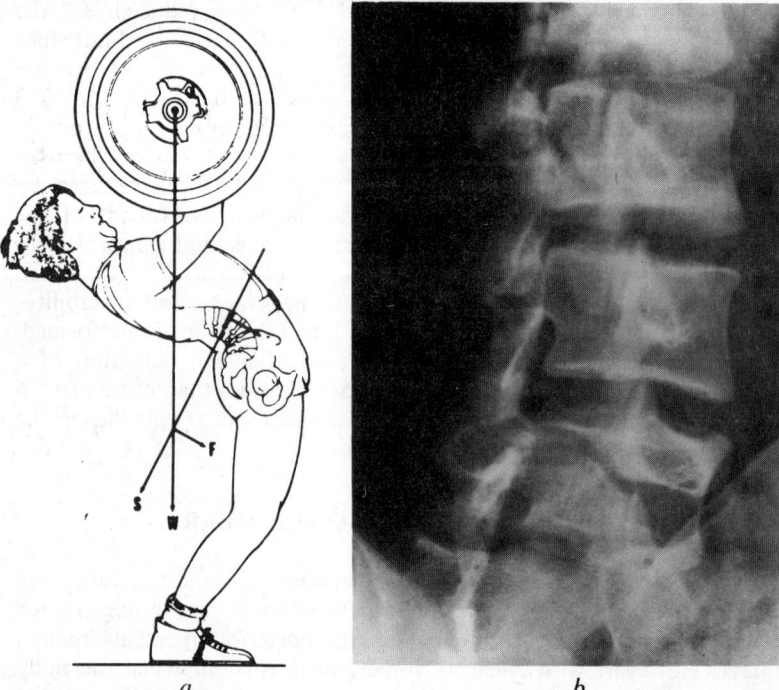

Fig. 63. *a*, Exaggerated 'lean-back' during the press, with a force tending to displace L5 anteriorly and causing considerable shearing forces resisted by the pars interarticularis. (W = weight, S = shear, F = resultant.) (Troup, 1970.) *b*, The defect in pes interarticularis (spondylolysis) is clearly seen on an oblique radiograph of a professional footballer.

stretcher. If there is no cord injury the patient is treated with 6–12 weeks of bed rest and, if needed, plaster immobilization. During this period spontaneous interbody fusion will occur due to the bony damage. When a good closed reduction cannot be achieved or if the damage is mainly ligamentous then surgical reduction and internal fixation are used. With a fixation device is wise to apply a bone graft because ligament repair will not be sufficient to prevent late displacement.

SPONDYLOLYSIS
Spondylolysis is a break in the continuity of the pars interarticularis of the neural arch almost always in the lumbar spine. Although it has been considered to be a congenital defect it is probably a stress fracture in athletes. It is not uncommon in soccer players (defenders who head the ball frequently), fast bowlers, American football linemen (Ferguson, 1974), oarsmen, weight-lifters (*Fig.* 63), and javelin and

hammer throwers. Although it may be asymptomatic it usually produces lumbar pain referred to the buttocks and legs. Sometimes players complain of lower abdominal discomfort especially in the region of the rectus abdominis insertion. A radiograph may show a unilateral or bilateral lesion.

Treatment
Rest, analgesics and a plaster or lumbar support are effective but there must be an adequate period off play to allow the symptoms to subside, usually 2–3 months are required. Like all stress fractures the lesion will heal but faults in technique need rectifying. If the condition is bilateral and there is forward slip of the upper vertebral body the defect may only heal by fibrous tissue and a spondylolisthesis has resulted.

SPONDYLOLISTHESIS
There is usually a slip of L4 on L5 or L5 on S1. Symptoms are aggravated by exercise and radiate to the buttocks and legs. In 5 per cent of cases there may be a disc lesion as well. This fact should not be forgotten.

Clinical examination may reveal paraspinal muscle spasm and tight hamstrings with a marked dimpling of the skin over the slipped spinous process. An anteroposterior radiograph will show that the upper border of the involved vertebra is too low, i.e. on a level with the transverse process. Lateral views will demonstrate a forward shift, a gap in the pars interarticularis or an elongated lamina and defective facets. Oblique views and radiological screening may show the defect more clearly than a plain lateral film.

Treatment
Conservative treatment (as described *above*) may be used if the symptoms are mild.

The principal methods of surgical treatment are:
1. Buck (1970) regarded the bony gap as a fatigue fracture and advised direct repair, providing that there is little vertebral slipping. The fibrous tissue is excised exposing the defect and the bone ends are trimmed. Then the area is transfixed with a screw and cancellous bone chips added. Both sides are treated. The player stays in bed for only a few days and begins light training at 4 weeks. Buck reports a return to football in 12 weeks.
2. Intertransverse grafting of the slipped vertebra to the one below can be performed.
3. The bony defect can be grafted with cancellous bone.

Following a bone fusion operation ((2) and (3)), the player lies prone in bed for 4–6 weeks, and can then get up in a plaster jacket for 4–8 weeks. A lumbosacral support can be used in the latter period of mobilization as an additional safeguard when the jacket has been discarded. Sport can begin at 6–12 months but training must be gradual in the early stages and all weight-training, if it involves lifting or carrying, forbidden. The rapid return to sport (within 12 weeks or so) after the Buck procedure makes it the treatment of choice; also following this operation a plaster jacket is not usually required.

BACKACHE
The commonest causes of backache in sportsmen are ligamentous strain, muscle injury, degeneration of the lower lumbar facets, a prolapsed intervertebral disc, a compression fracture, sacralization of the lumbar vertebra, mild scoliosis, spina bifida and dysraphism, spinal stenosis, spondylolysis and spondylolisthesis.

Prolapsed Intervertebral Disc
This condition is common in the lumbar region especially at L4–5 and L5–S1 levels. Mild cases need rest (3 weeks), analgesics and physiotherapy; moderate cases need an epidural injection. When there is nerve root compression with absent reflexes, reduced sensation and muscle power the player is best treated for 4 weeks with a plaster jacket, or, if mobility exacerbates the pain, traction in hospital for 2–3 weeks. If there is no response to conservative measures the author favours a myelogram and if a disc protrusion is found a fenestration laminectomy is performed. Even in the absence of clear-cut clinical signs two adjacent levels should be explored since an associated smaller disc protrusion may be masked by a larger herniated disc at a higher or lower level.

Back injuries can be a problem for many years and it is important that once they have settled acute exacerbations are not allowed to occur. Physiotherapy should include strengthening the abdominal muscles as well as the spinal muscles, the former (oblique muscles) can be looked on as the 'guy ropes' of the spine. Training with heavy weights and on hard gym floors should be restricted or forbidden. Care should be taken in choosing athletic shoes without too high a heel and to ensure that studding is such that most of the pivoting occurs on the forefoot and not at the heel where it will be transmitted to the lumbar spine. A single pivot stud can be placed anteriorly with four shorter studs (two sole/two heel) behind. After a fenestration laminectomy training can begin at 4–6 weeks and match play at 8–12 weeks in most instances.

Chapter 13

Chest, abdomen and pelvic injuries

These injuries occur in contact sports, after high-speed accidents in motor sports and in horse-riding. The more serious demand urgent specialist advice and treatment, their early diagnosis being the prerogative of the sports doctor. Marathon runners may develop benign haematuria, clearing within 48 hours of a race.

CHEST INJURIES
Soft-tissue bruising and rib fractures are common in soccer, rugby and boxing. A fracture of the ribs can be best treated by analgesics and breathing exercises; strapping is detrimental to lung excursion. Multiple rib fractures may produce a flail segment. Rib fractures may sometimes be difficult to see on a chest radiograph and the number seen may be fewer than exist. The lung should be inspected for contusion and a pneumothorax sought on the anteroposterior film. Occasionally stress fractures of the ribs are produced in tennis and rowing. These respond to rest. Tears of the pectoralis major and minor may occur with excessive pushing or lifting (gymnastics, weight-lifting) and tenderness is found over the insertions on the ribs or sternal junction. Disorders of the thoracic spine can cause radiation of pain around the chest wall. A small haematoma or an area of fat necrosis may be found after breast trauma in a woman; however, other more serious conditions may have to be excluded by biopsy.

Lung Injury
The lung may suffer contusion and a small haemoptysis result. A radiograph shows an area of consolidation. Prophylactic antibiotics are given and the player rested for several days. Sport can be resumed

in 2 weeks in most cases. In more serious accidents the opposite lung may be affected (*contre-coup* effect) as well and a mixture of oedema, interstitial haemorrhage, atelectasis and alveolar haemorrhage is responsible for the radiological appearance. Such serious injuries may need intermittent positive-pressure respiration (Keen, 1975).

Subcutaneous Emphysema
This follows an escape of air from a damaged lung or air passage which then finds its way into the chest wall, mediastinum and subcutaneous tissues by way of a tear in the parietal pleura. It is occasionally associated with an open chest wound; and when there is a rapid accumulation a torn bronchus should be suspected.

TREATMENT
No specific treatment is required for the subcutaneous emphysema but attention should be directed to treating the underlying cause.

Pneumothorax
This follows damage to the lung or air passages; rarely is the oesophagus responsible. It may be small or large, unilateral or bilateral. In young people rib fractures may not be present and trauma may not be a significant feature. The author has seen this condition in a university rugby player effecting a touch-down, the principal complaint being a sudden chest pain while sprinting for the line.

A small amount of air will readily absorb but larger amounts may cause lung collapse or compressive effects (tension pneumothorax). Increasing dyspnoea, chest pain, a resonance on percussion and absent breath sounds on the affected side are found. In an emergency a wide-bore needle is inserted into the pleural space at the area of maximal resonance. Keen (1975) stresses the importance of a preliminary radiograph before such treatment unless the situation is urgent for in the absence of radiological confirmation serious mischief can be done. An intercostal catheter drainage system is connected to an underwater seal; the safest and most reliable site being the second intercostal space anteriorly in the midclavicular line. Sport can begin after 3 months.

Haemothorax
Usually found with a pneumothorax the bleeding is commonly from the intercostal, internal mammary and diaphragmatic vessels. Since each pleural cavity can contain 3 litres of blood a careful check must be made on the pulse and blood pressure if this injury is suspected. A small haemothorax causes few, if any, symptoms. Radiologically there may be a loss of the acute costophrenic angle together with a

hazy appearance over the lower chest. Since as much as 500 ml of blood can be hidden behind the dome of the diaphragm the radiological assessment of blood loss is difficult. Treatment is by aspiration but with large bleeds tube drainage and an underwater seal are required. Thoracotomy is only needed in the most serious cases.

Lung Laceration
Lung lacerations do not bleed freely because of the low pulmonary arterial pressure; the treatment is as for pneumothorax and haemothorax if both coexist (Keen, 1975).

Cardiac Injury
Heart or great vessel injury can result from trauma to the chest. Contusion to the precordium can result in ECG changes, with ST segment depression and T wave inversion. Arrhythmias are not uncommon but usually transient. Treatment is by complete bed rest for several days and sport is not commenced for up to 3 months. A further ECG may be required before activity is resumed.

ABDOMINAL INJURY
Blows to the Abdomen
Direct blows to the abdomen rarely injure the contents because of the protection of the strong abdominal muscles and the mobility of many of the viscera. Relatively fixed organs are the most frequently damaged. Liver injury may follow a blow to the right lower ribs; a spleen may be injured with a blow on the left lower ribs. Kidneys, intestines, testes and urethra are also commonly damaged. In all cases localized pain, shock, abdominal rigidity and vomiting are found. Pain may be referred to the shoulders as the abdominal contents or blood irritates the diaphragm. Blood may appear in the urine or as a melaena.

TREATMENT
Mild contusion of the kidneys can be treated conservatively and a precautionary IVP taken. Other major abdominal trauma requires laparotomy and expert advice.

Haematomas and Sprains
Haematomas and sprains of the abdominal wall are of minor importance and heal with rest for 1–2 weeks. Sprains of the pelvic insertion of rectus abdominis may require local infiltration with hydrocortisone and lignocaine if they become chronically painful.

Hernias
These need surgical correction because of the dangers of strangulation in sportsmen; 6–12 weeks later sport can begin again.

PELVIC INJURIES

Fractures of the pelvis are divided into stable and unstable. Any pelvic injury may damage the contained viscera and in this respect urethral damage is of particular importance. No clinical examination of the pelvis should exclude an examination of the external urethral meatus for blood. Injury to the bladder, bowel and genitalia (male and female) may coexist. In serious fractures blood loss should be assessed by careful observation of pulse and blood pressure, a loss of 2 litres or more is not unknown after major pelvic fractures, and if branches of the internal iliac are involved bleeding can be greater than this amount.

If damage to the urethra is suspected the player must not pass urine until urgent advice is obtained from a genito-urinary surgeon.

Simple stable fractures are treated by bed rest for 1–4 weeks and then mobilization depending on the severity of the injury; unstable fractures are treated by reduction through skeletal traction or a lumbosacral corset depending on whether the injury is caused by a vertical force or a hinge force. Three months of non-weight-bearing are advocated.

Avulsion Fractures

Violent muscle action in an athletic adolescent may avulse a traction epiphysis. The muscles concerned are the sartorius, rectus femoris (*Fig.* 64) and the hamstrings.

DIAGNOSIS

The site of the avulsion is tender and a radiograph defines the lesion.

TREATMENT

Reduction is unnecessary. The patient is rested for a few days with the injured muscle in a relaxed position of comfort. Then normal activities are resumed. Sport begins after 4 weeks or so depending on local discomfort.

Strains

Hamstring origin strains are common in sprinters and footballers and the sudden severe pain in the buttock may mimic sciatica. Tenderness is found over the hamstring's insertion. Treatment is by heat, and gentle stretching under local anaesthesia. A similar *adductor origin strain* (rider's strain) is found in cyclists, horsemen and horsewomen, runners, footballers and fast bowlers. Pain and stiffness are felt in the groin and there is local tenderness and pain on abduction. Treatment is by manipulation under general anaesthesia, massage or local steroids. Calcification in the adductor longus tendon is seen in horse riders and may require local excision; usually heat and analgesics are helpful

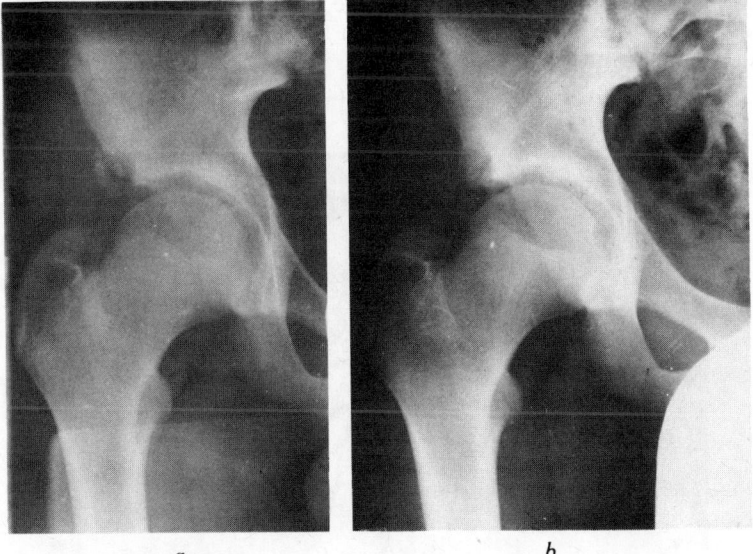

Fig. 64. *a*, Avulsion fracture at the anterior inferior iliac spine in a hurdler aged 15 years. *b*, Treated by rest and limited activity for 4 weeks.

during an acutely painful episode. The breast stroke in swimming, with its unusual leg action, may produce chronic adductor tendinitis.

Fractures of the Sacrum and Coccyx
These are usually not displaced and simply require analgesics. However, sitting may require a sorbo-rubber cushion for several weeks. Chronic pain after a fracture in this region is treated by local anaesthetic injections; persistent coccygeal tenderness may warrant excision of the coccyx.

Osteitis Pubis
This is usually a self-limiting condition of sportsmen, often in their thirties, and common in professional footballers, but may be found in runners and long-distance walkers

DIAGNOSIS
The earliest symptom is discomfort in the groin, of gradual onset after exercise, exacerbated by sprinting, jumping and striding widely. Gradually the pain extends over the whole of the pubic area, perineum and down the inner aspect of the thighs (along the distribution of the obturator nerve). Tenderness is found over the symphysis, the whole

of the pubic bone, on compressing the pelvis, on full flexion of either leg, on passive abduction at the hips and on resisted contraction of the adductor muscles of the thighs.

The histology is depicted in *Fig. 65a*.

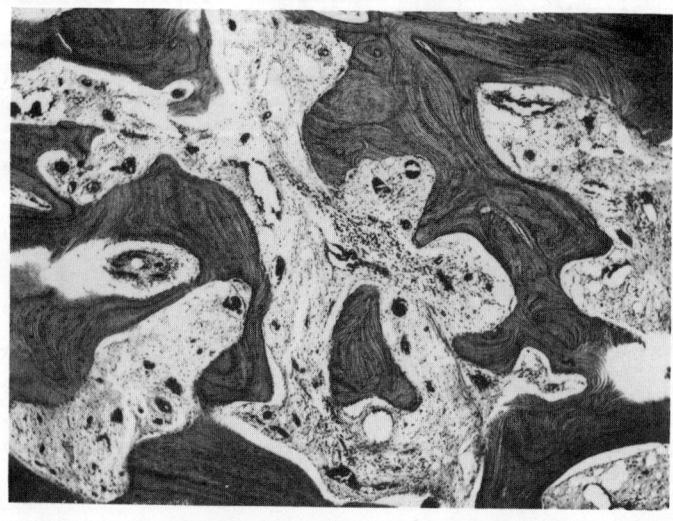

a

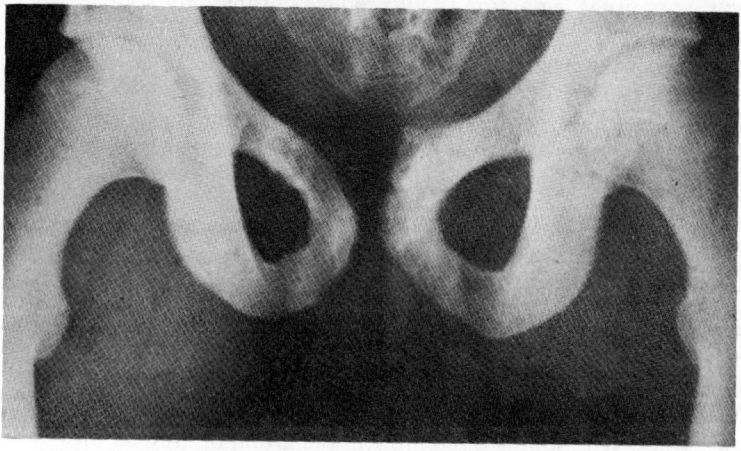

b

Fig. 65. *a*, Histology of osteitis pubis showing active bone resorption, fibrosis of marrow space, increased vascularity and collections of chronic inflammatory cells; *b*, Radiology (*see text*).

A radiograph (*Fig.* 65*b*) shows fraying of the corners of the symphysis, fluffiness of its margins, elevation of the periosteum in relation to muscle attachments, osteoporosis and 'moth-eaten' erosions of the affected medial parts of the pubic bodies and inferior rami, widening of the symphysis and, in severe cases, instability with the opposing surfaces moving 6–12 mm (Adams and Chandler, 1953).

Laboratory investigations are unhelpful and urinalysis is usually normal but a urinary infection must be excluded, particularly prostatitis and Reiter's disease. Ankylosing spondylitis must also be remembered as a possible cause of inguinocrural pain. Sometimes narrowing of the hip joints may be found in association with osteitis pubis.

TREATMENT

All activity stops during the acute phase which may last for 4–8 weeks. During the first month anti-inflammatory drugs are given and shortwave diathermy may be of value in the later stages. After 2 months radiographs show early recalcification and gentle mobilization and running are begun. Full sport is resumed at 3 months in most cases. Within a year the radiological changes disappear apart from some patchy osteosclerosis and spurs from periosteal new bone formation at muscle attachments.

Bacteria are not implicated in the aetiology (Wiltse and Frantz, 1956). The blood supply of the pubic bones arises mainly from a periosteal plexus and is through loops that are essentially end-arteries. Trauma, direct or indirect through constant muscle strain, causes periosteal and subperiosteal damage and subsequent thrombosis of the end-vessels thus producing aseptic necrosis of bone and fibrocartilage. Harris and Murray (1974) found that 76 per cent of professional players in one soccer club showed some changes on routine pelvic radiographs. In a review of 37 athletes with this condition they stressed the fact that spontaneous remissions occur with rest and that stabilization of the pubic symphysis with bone-block grafts was rarely needed.

Refractory cases may take 9–12 months to become symptom-free, although most players return in 6 months. It is important not to overtreat this condition with numerous local injections and a zealous use of shortwave diathermy or ultrasound—thus hindering the natural healing process.

Chapter 14

Injuries to the skin

Lacerations and abrasions are very common injuries, often requiring treatment during the course of a sports event. In most instances the player can resume playing unless some important structure such as a ligament, vessel, nerve, etc. is involved.

It is a matter of common experience that wounds heal best when healthy tissue lies in close contact—undisturbed by movement and infection. In contrast, contused or jagged wounds need surgical intervention and the excision of the necrotic tissue. For superficial cuts that are not liable to disturbance apposition is obtained by adhesive plaster or tape (such as dumb-bell sutures or Steritape). In areas subject to movement, or in large wounds, nylon, black silk and dexon can be used.

EXPLORATION AND REPAIR
All deep wounds should be gently explored under either a general or local anaesthetic to see what important structures are involved. Foreign bodies such as soil, grass and grit are removed by gentle lavage with sterile saline. Occasionally the wound may have to be enlarged and this should be planned with due regard for flexure lines and the possible risk of endangering the capillary circulation in the skin flaps or wound edges.

Toilet of Wounds
Dead and damaged tissues are completely excised; fascia, fat and fibrous tissues (tendons, ligaments, etc.) are trimmed and the skin edges are cut to linear surfaces with good capillary bleeding. Loose fragments of bone and cartilage are discarded unless their size, structural importance or soft-tissue attachments make it preferable to

retain them. All muscle that does not bleed requires excision but bruised muscle with a good circulation is saved.

Repair
Skin suture should always be carried out in good lighting conditions. Local anaesthesia is commonly used by club doctors, but direct infiltration of dirty or contused wounds is not recommended since bacteria may be spread to the adjacent tissues. In these cases a regional block or general anaesthesia (in hospital) is preferred. Nylon or similar analogues are best since they are less liable than black silk to act as a nidus for infection. A subcutaneous stitch with dexon can be employed in facial lacerations, in children's wounds, or when a plaster has to be employed for several weeks. Primary repair is not carried out if there is serious doubt about the viability of the remaining tissues, if infection is suspected, if there has been a delay of over 6 hours, or if there is excessive swelling. Secondary suture and skin grafting can be carried out later.

When there is doubt about the complexity of the laceration, especially in young children, general anaesthesia should be used.

Antibiotics
If adequate excision of devitalized tissue has been performed then prophylactic antibiotics are not needed. However, when required, there is a wide choice of local antibiotics which can be used either alone or in combination. Polymyxin, neomycin and bacitracin are available in spray or powder form; while hibitane, cetrimide and noxyflex are available as solutions. Intramuscular penicillin is effective against most strains of clostridia (tetanus and gas gangrene) and streptococcus; oral penicillin V can be substituted after 24 hours. The author favours a combination of flucloxacillin and talampicillin. If other antibiotics are required (e.g. sulphonamides, streptomycin, fusidic acid, erythromycin and the cephalosporins) there should be good clinical and bacteriological evidence; using antibiotics to their best advantage calls for both discrimination and restraint.

Tetanus Immunization
All sportsmen, especially contact sports players, should be immunized against tetanus. The date of immunization should be recorded on the player's chart. A non-immune player receives an immediate dose of 0·5 ml of tetanus vaccine (toxoid) and booster doses at 6 weeks and 6 months. Immunity is maintained with 3-yearly doses.

Infections
When there is a spreading skin infection (often from a dirty stud mark in the tibial region) antibiotics are given and the area can be rested

in a plaster-of-Paris. The period of immobilization is very effective and it is worth noting that in one season with a professional soccer club the author used more lower limb plasters to help contain infection than were applied for ligamentous injuries.

Surgery is required to release an abscess and remove foreign or dead tissues.

WOUNDS ON THE SCALP AND FACE
A special mention must be made of wounds in these areas since they are common in contact sports and often require immediate treatment so that the player can continue with the match. Small cuts can be approximated with adhesive skin sutures but the continued bleeding may cause them to become unstuck. As a rapid alternative one or two skin sutures of nylon or silk can be used for immediate approximation and an adhesive dressing applied. After the event the wound can be fully sutured. On the whole, the author favours immediate, accurate and complete suturing of any wound to minimize the dangers of infection and an ugly scar; even if this procedure means the player abandoning the event or a lengthy delay. Cuts crossing facial creases, on the eyelids and ears, and across the vermilion of the lips need careful suturing. Haematomas of the ear need aspiration or incision and a pressure dressing.

ABRASIONS
These readily heal but all particles of grass and grit must be removed; this can be done with a fine jet of sterile saline or a mild antiseptic solution. The area is covered with a plastic-spray covering or a non-stick dressing. A petroleum-jelly-impregnated dressing is used on the buttocks or thigh where chafing irritates the wound. 'Mat friction burns' are troublesome in wrestling.

BLISTERS
Blisters are the curse of the pre-season training; a consequence of unaccustomed activity and new, rigid equipment. They are produced by tangential skin stresses. Small blisters are covered with a small felt pad or adhesive dressing, but larger blisters are burst with a sterile needle and dressed. Surgical spirit or mercurochrome can be used to dry up weeping surfaces and harden skin. Boots, shoes, oars, rackets, etc. should be checked for friction areas, often minor ridges in the bindings or in the soles can cause blistering, and these faults can be rectified with soft padding. New shoes need running in slowly and as a rule an athlete requires two pairs of shoes or boots at a time—one pair wearing in, the other pair wearing out.

CARE OF TOE-NAILS

Footballers may miss up to 8 weeks of play with an ingrowing toe-nail and in the preparation for the World Cup the strictest attention was given to the care of the toe-nails and feet. Daily foot inspections were carried out and there was a demonstration on how to cut toe-nails, with details of how the smallest of sharp points from an incorrectly cut nail could lead to eventual infection (Muckle and Shepherdson, 1975). Toe-nails must be clean and cut horizontally and not allowed to become jagged.

Ingrowing toe-nails can be treated by padding between the toes (such as cotton-wool) to separate the great and second toe when the lesion is on this apposing surface. Antibiotics do not help and once a granuloma has developed it requires excision with either trimming of the nail or, perhaps, partial or complete nail avulsion.

FUNGAL INFECTIONS

Players are prone to fungal infections between the toes ('athlete's foot') and in the groin; these infections are transmitted in communal baths, and therefore showers are to be preferred. Antifungal creams containing undecylenic acid, miconazole and clotrimazole are usually prescribed. Sometimes the long-term administration of griseofulvin is needed but a dermatologist should be consulted first. In the author's experience gentian violet still proves to be efficacious in resistant cases.

To help eliminate an infection within a club, strict attention to personal hygiene, showers and the regular washing of equipment (stockings, shorts, etc.) must be observed. Players must be dissuaded from using each others' towels and sports clothes.

References

ADAMS S. (1980) Ibuprofen: pharmokinetics. *Br. J. Clin. Practice* Suppl. 6, 3.
ADAMS R. J. and CHANDLER F. A. (1953) Osteitis pubis of traumatic aetiology. *J. Bone Joint Surg.* 35A, 685.
ALLEMANDOU A. (1976) A statistical review of injuries. In *Injuries in Rugby Football and other Team Sports*. Dublin, Irish Rugby Football Union.
ALM A., LAMKE L. O. and LILJEDAHL S. O. (1975) Surgical treatment of dislocation of the peroneal tendons. *Injury* 7, 14.
ANDERSEN, N. H. and RAMWELL, P. W. (1974) Biological aspects of prostaglandins. *Arch. Intern. Med.* 133, 30.
BARBER H. M. (1973) Horse-play: survey of accidents with horses. *Br. Med. J.* 3, 532.
BATEMAN J. E. (1969). Shoulder injuries in throwing sports. In *Symposium on Sports Medicine*. St Louis, Mosby.
BEARDEN J. M., HUGHSTON J. C. and WHATLEY G. S. (1973) Acromioclavicular dislocation, methods of treatment. *J. Sports Med.* 1, 4.
BEHLING F. (1973) Treatment of acromioclavicular separations. *Orthop. Clin. North Am.* 4, 747.
BLAZINA M. E. (1966) Shoulder injuries in athletes. *J. Am. Coll. Health Assoc.* 15, 143.
BLAZINA M. E. (1973) Jumper's knee. *Orthop. Clin. North Am.* 4, 67.
BLONSTEIN J. L. (1960) Electroencephalography in boxers. *J. Sports Med. Phys. Fitness* 1, 30.
BLONSTEIN J. L. (1966) Medical aspects of amateur boxing. *Proc. R. Soc. Med.* 59, 649.
BLONSTEIN J. L. and SCHMID L. (1974) Causes of death in ex-boxers. *Br. J. Sports Med.* 8, 205.
BLUMENKRANTZ N. and SØNDERGAARD J. (1972) Effects of prostaglandin E_1 $F_{1\alpha}$ on the biosynthesis of collagen. *Nature (New Biol.)* 239, 246.
BOURNE M. and BENTLEY S. (1980) Enhanced recovery from sports injuries. *Br J. Clin. Practice* Suppl. 6, 72.
BOYD H. B. and ANDERSON L. D. (1961) A method for reinsertion of the distal biceps brachii tendon. *J. Bone Joint Surg.* 43A, 1041.
BUCK J. E. (1970) Direct repair of the defect in spondylolisthesis. *J. Bone Joint Surg.* 52B, 432.
CAVE E. F. and ROWE C. R. (1947) Bankart operation. *Surg. Clin. North Am.* 27, 1289.
CHO K. O. (1975) Reconstruction of the anterior cruciate ligament by semitendinosus tendon. *J. Bone Joint Surg.* 57A, 608.
COLLINS H. R. and WILDE A. H. (1973) Shoulder instability in athletes. *Orthop. Clin. North Am.* 4, 759.
CRAIG R. P. (1975) The quantitative evaluation of the use of oral proteolytic enzymes in the treatment of sprained ankles. *Injury* 6, 313.

REFERENCES

CRANE J., GIBSON T. and BUSSON M. (1980) A comparative study of ibuprofen and indomethacin in ligamentous injuries of the ankle. *Br. J. Clin. Practice* Suppl. 6, 92.
CRENSHAW A. H. (1971) *Campbell's Operative Orthopaedics*. St Louis, Mosby.
CRENSHAW A. H. and KILGORE W. E. (1966) Surgical treatment of bicipital tenosynovitis. *J. Bone Joint Surg.* **48A**, 1496.
CROMPTON B. A. and TUBBS N. (1977) A survey of sports injuries in Birmingham. *Br. J. Sports Med.* **11**, 12.
DANDY D. J. and JACKSON R. W. (1975) The diagnosis of problems after meniscectomy. *J. Bone Joint Surg.* **57B**, 349.
DEVAS M. B. (1969) Stress fractures in athletes. *Proc. R. Soc. Med.* **62**, 933.
DEXEL M. and SCHREIBER A. (1979) Diagnosis of the unstable knee joint. *Ital. J. Sp. Traumatology* **1**, 13.
DUNLOP J. (1939) Transcondylar fractures of the humerus in childhood. *J. Bone Joint Surg.* **21**, 59.
DURBIN F. C. (1957) Fracture-dislocation of the cervical spine. *J. Bone Joint Surg.* **39B**, 23.
DUVRIES H. L. (1959) *Surgery of the Foot*. St Louis, Mosby.
ECKERT W. R. and DAVIES E. A. jun. (1976) Acute rupture of the peroneal retinaculum. *J. Bone Joint Surg.* **58A**, 670.
ERIKSSON E. (1976) Symposium on ski trauma and skiing safety. *Orthop. Clin. North Am.* **7**, 3.
FERGUSON R. J. (1974) Low back pain in college football linemen. *J. Bone Joint Surg.* **56A**, 1300.
FLATT A. E. (1969) Athletic injuries of the hand. In *Symposium of Sports Medicine*. St Louis, Mosby.
FLYNN M. and KELLY J. P. (1976) Local excision of cyst of lateral meniscus of the knee without recurrence. *J. Bone Joint Surg.* **58B**, 88.
GARFIELD J. (1973) In *Trauma Surgery* (ed. Powley P.). Bristol, Wright.
GEAR M. W. L. (1967) The late results of meniscectomy. *Br. J. Surg.* **54**, 270.
GOLDBERG B., WITMAN P. A., GLEIM G. W. and NICHOLAS J. A. (1979) Children's sports injuries. *Phys. Sportsmed.* **7**, 93.
GOOD C. J., JONES M. A. and LIVINGSTONE B. N. (1975) Reconstruction of the lateral ligament of the ankle. *Injury* **7**, 63.
HARRIS N. H. and MURRAY R. G. (1974) Lesions of the symphysis pubis in athletes. *J. Bone Joint Surg.* **56B**, 563.
HEPPENSTALL R. B. (1975) Fractures and dislocations of the distal clavicle. *Orthop. Clin. North Am.* **6**, 477.
HUGHSTON J. C., ANDERSON J. R., CROSS M. J. and MOSCHI A. (1976) Classification of knee ligament instabilities. Part 1: The medial compartment and cruciate ligaments. *J. Bone Joint Surg.* **58A**, 159.
HUSKISSON E. C., BERRY H., STREET F. G. and MEDHURST H. E. (1973) Indomethacin for soft-tissue injuries. *Rheum Rehab.* **12**, 159.
INGLIS A. E., SCOTT N. W., SCULO T. T. and PATTERSON A. H. (1975) Rupture of the tendo Achillis: an objective assessment of non-surgical and surgical treatment. *J. Bone Joint Surg.* **57A**, 1172.
INSALL J., FALVO K. A. and WISE D. W. (1976) Chondromalacia patellae. *J. Bone Joint Surg.* **58A**, 1.
ISMAIL A. M., BALAKRISHNAN R. and RAJAKUMAR M. K. (1969) Rupture of patellar ligament after steroid injection. *J. Bone Joint Surg.* **51B**, 503.
JACKSON D. W. (1976) Chronic rotator cuff impingement in the throwing athlete. *Am. J. Sports Med.* **4**, 231.
JACKSON J. P. (1967) Degenerative changes in the knee after meniscectomy. *J. Bone Joint Surg.* **49B**, 584.

REFERENCES

JOHANSEN O. (1955) In *Sports Injuries*. Oslo.
JOHNSON R. J., POPE M. H. and ETTLINGER C. (1976) Inter-relationship between ski accidents, the resultant injury, the skier's characteristics, and the ski boot binding system. *Orthop. Clin. North Am.* **7**, 11.
KEEN G. (1975) *Chest Injuries*. Bristol, Wright.
KENWRIGHT J. K. and TAYLOR R. G. (1970). Major injuries of the talus. *J. Bone Joint Surg.* **52B**, 36.
KILLEY H. C. (1968) Maxillo-facial injuries. *Br. J. Hosp. Med.* **2**, 917.
KYLE J. W. (1976) Cervical spine injuries. In *Injuries in Rugby Football and other Team Sports*. Dublin, Irish Rugby Football Union, p. 116.
LA CAVA G. (1960) *Indagine Clinico Stastica sulle Lesioni Traumatische da Sport*. Turin, Edizioni Minerva Medica.
LEA E. B. and SMITH L. (1972) Non-surgical treatment of tendo Achillis rupture. *J. Bone Joint Surg.* **54A**, 1398.
LEACH R. E., O'CONNOR P. and JONES R. (1979) Acromionectomy for tendinitis of the shoulder in athletes. *Phys. Sportsmed.* **7**, 96.
LECLERC F. P. and AUTISSIER D. (1969) The use of indomethacin in the treatment of limb injuries and their sequelae. *Gaz. Hôp. Paris* **1**, 31.
LINDHOLM A. (1959) A new method of operation in subcutaneous rupture of the Achilles tendon. *Acta Chir. Scand.* **117**, 261.
LOMBARDO S. T., KERLAN R. K., JOBE F. W., CARTER V. S., BLAZINA M. E. and SHIELDS C. L. jun. (1976) The modified Bristow procedure for recurrent dislocation of the shoulder. *J. Bone Joint Surg.* **58A**, 256.
LYNN T. A. (1966) Repair of torn Achilles tendon using the plantaris tendon as a reinforcing membrane. *J. Bone Joint Surg.* **48A**, 268.
MCGLASHAN T. P. L. (1976) Current thinking on mouth guards. In *Injuries in Rugby Football and other Team Sports*. Dublin, Irish Rugby Football Union, p. 147.
MCLATCHIE G. R. (1979) Surgical and orthopaedic problems in sport karate. *Medisport* **1**, 40.
MCLAUGHLIN H. L. (1947) Repair of major tendon ruptures by buried removable sutures. *Am. J. Surg.* **74**, 758.
MAGNUSON P. B. and STACK J. K. (1943) Recurrent dislocation of the shoulder. *JAMA* **123**, 889.
MILLER J. E. (1960) Javelin thrower's elbow. *J. Bone Joint Surg.* **42B**, 788.
MORREY B. F. and JANES J. M. (1976) Recurrent anterior dislocation of the shoulder. *J. Bone Joint Surg.* **58A**, 252.
MORRIS M. (1963) A sports injury survey of Greater Birmingham. *Phys. Educ.* **55**, 41
MUCKLE D. S. (1972a) Shoulder injuries in sport. *Br. J. Sports Med.* **6**, 77.
MUCKLE D. S. (1972b) Intra-articular ganglion of the knee. *J. Bone Joint Surg* **54B**, 520.
MUCKLE D. S. (1973) Dislocation of the superior tibiofibular joint. *Br. J. Sports Med.* **7**, 365.
MUCKLE D. S. (1974) Comparative study of ibuprofen and aspirin in soft tissue injuries. *Rheum. Rehab.* **13**, 141.
MUCKLE D. S. (1976) First aid in sport. *Mod. Med.* **21**, 44.
MUCKLE D. S. (1977) A double-blind trial of flurbiprofen and aspirin in soft-tissue trauma. *Rheum. Rehab.* **16**, 58.
MUCKLE D. S. (1980a) Osteoarthrosis of the knee following meniscectomy. M.D. Thesis. Univ. Newcastle.
MUCKLE D. S. (1980b) Ibuprofen in soft tissue injuries—a long-term clinical evaluation. *Br. J. Clin. Practice* Suppl. 6, 71.
MUCKLE D. S. and MINNS R. J. (1979) The use of filamentous carbon fibre for the repair of osteoarthritic articular cartilage. *J. Bone Joint Surg.* **61B**, 381.

REFERENCES

MUCKLE D. S. and SHEPHERDSON H. (1975) *Football Fitness and Injuries.* London, Pelham.

MÜLLER M. E., ALLGÖWER M. and WILLENEGGER H. W. (1970) *Manual of Internal Fixation.* Berlin, Springer-Verlag.

NICHOLAS J. A. (1973a) Injuries to the menisci of the knees. *Orthop. Clin. North Am.* **4**, 647.

NICHOLAS J. A. (1973b) The five-one reconstruction for anteromedial instability of the knee. *J. Bone Joint Surg.* **55A**, 899.

NICHOLAS J. A. (1974) Ankle injuries in athletes. *Orthop. Clin. North Am.* **5**, 153.

NOBLE J. and HAMBLEN D. L. (1975) The pathology of the degenerate meniscus lesion. *J. Bone Joint Surg.* **57B**, 180.

ORAVA S. and PURANEN J. (1979) Athlete's leg pains. *Br. J. Sports Med.* **13**, 92.

O'DONOGHUE D. H. (1973) Treatment of acute ligamentous injuries of the knee. *Orthop. Clin. North Am.* **4**, 617.

OSMOND-CLARKE H. (1948) Habitual dislocation of the shoulder—the Putti–Platt operation. *J. Bone Joint Surg.* **30B**, 19.

RITTER M. A. and GOSLING C. (1980) *The Knee: A Guide to the Examination and Diagnosis of Ligament Injuries.* Springfield, Ill., Thomas.

ROBERTS R. R. (1963) Triservice Medical Survey on Shoulder Dislocation. Dept., Navy.

ROLES N. C. and MAUDSLEY R. H. (1972) Radial tunnel syndrome: resistant tennis elbow as a nerve entrapment. *J. Bone Joint Surg.* **54B**, 499.

ROTHMAN R. H., MARVEL J. P. jun. and HEPPENSTALL R. B. (1975) Recurrent anterior dislocation of the shoulder. *Orthop. Clin. North Am.* **6**, 417.

ROWE N. L. and KILLEY H. C. (1968) *Fractures of the Facial Skeleton*, 2nd ed. Edinburgh, Livingstone.

SALTER R. B. and HARRIS W. R. (1963) Injuries involving the epiphyseal plate. *J. Bone Joint Surg.* **45A**, 587.

SCOTT J. C. and ORR M. M. (1973) Injuries of the acromioclavicular joint. *Injury* **5**, 13.

SHEPHARD R. J. (1974) Sudden death—a significant hazard of exercise. *Br. J. Sports Med.* **8**, 101.

SLOCUM D. B. and LARSON R. L. (1968) Pes anserinus transplantation. *J. Bone Joint Surg.* **50A**, 226.

SLOCUM D. B. and JAMES S. (1968) Biomechanics of running. *J.A.M.A.* **205**, 721.

SLOCUM D. B., LARSON R. L. and JAMES S. L. (1973) Late reconstruction procedures used to stabilize the knee. *Orthop. Clin. North Am.* **4**, 679.

SMILLIE I. S. (1969) Knee injuries in athletes. *Proc. R. Soc. Med.* **62**, 937.

SMILLIE I. S. (1973) *Injuries of the Knee Joint*, 4th ed. Edinburgh, Churchill-Livingstone.

SOEUR R. and REMY R. (1975) Fractures of the calcaneus with displacement of the thalmic portion. *J. Bone Joint Surg.* **57B**, 413.

SPERRYN P. N. (1973) Traumatic bursitis in a boxer's hand. *Br. J. Sports Med.* **7**, 103.

SUBOTNICK S. (1975) *Podiatric Sports Medicine.* New York, Futura Co.

TAPPER E. M. and HOOVER N. W. (1969) Late results after meniscectomy. *J. Bone Joint Surg.* **51A**, 517.

TROUP J. D. G. (1970) The risk of weight-training and weight-lifting in young people. *Br. J. Sports Med.* **5**, 27.

TUCKER W. E. and ARMSTRONG J. R. (1964) *Injury in Sport.* London, Staples Press.

VALTONEN E. J. and BUSSON M. (1978) A comparative study on ibuprofen and indomethacin in non-articular rheumatism. *Scand J. Rheum.* **7**, 183.

VAN MARION W. F. (1973) Indomethacin in the treatment of soft tissue lesions. *J. Int. Med. Res.* **1**, 151.

REFERENCES

WEBER B. G. (1966) Die Verletzungen des oberen Sprungglenkes. *Aktuelle Probleme in der Chirurgie*, Bd. 3. Bern and Stuttgart, Hüber.

WEIGHTMAN D. and BROWNE R. C. (1974) Injuries in rugby and association football. *Br. J. Sports Med.* **8**, 183.

WEIGHTMAN D. and BROWNE R. C. (1975) Injuries in eleven selected sports. *Br. J. Sports Med.* **9**, 136.

WILLIAMS J. G. P. (1976) Injuries of the lower limbs. In *Sports Medicine* (ed. Williams J. G. P. and Sperryn P.). London, Arnold. p. 428.

WILTSE L. L. and FRANTZ C. H. (1956) Non-suppurative osteitis pubis in the female. *J. Bone Joint Surg.* **38A**, 500.

ZADIK F. R. (1950) Obliteration of the nail bed of the great toe without shortening the terminal phalanx. *J. Bone Joint Surg.* **32B**, 66.

Index

Abdominal injuries, 141
Abrasions, 148
Accessory ossicles: foot, 96
Achilles tendon: chronic lesions, 43
Achilles tendon rupture, 29
Acromioclavicular dislocation, 101
Acromioclavicular subluxation, 101
Adductor strain: pelvis, 142
Ankle: chronic problems, 45, 88
   fractures, 91
   injuries, 86
   lateral ligament injuries, 88
   ligament tears, 88
   sprains, 87
Anterior chamber haemorrhages, 127
Anterior compartment syndromes, 42
Anterior thigh pain, 41
Antibiotics, 147
Assessment of head and spinal injuries, 15
Assessment of nerve and vascular damage, 13
Avulsion injuries: pelvis, 142

Backache, 138
Bailey procedure, 102
Bankart operation, 107
Baseball elbow, 38
Bennett's fracture, 115
Biceps tendon: dislocation, 24
   rupture, 24, 118
   tendinitis, 24
Blisters, 148
Boxer's knuckle, 120
Brain injury, 121
Bristow operation, 106
Bruised heel, 45
Bursae, 41

Capsulitis: shoulder, 118
Cardiac injury, 141
Cervical spine injuries, 133
Chest injuries, 139

Chondromalacia patellae, 51
Coccyx fracture, 143
Corneal abrasions, 126

De Quervain's tenovaginitis, 119
Dislocations: *see under area*

Ear injuries, 127
Elbow fractures and dislocations, 110
Elbow strains, 23, 37
Emergency treatment, 12
Epiphysial injuries, 102
Epistaxis, 129
Extradural bleeding, 122
Eye: foreign bodies, 126
   haematomas, 126
   injuries, 126
   injury prevention, 127

Facial fractures, 129
Facial injuries, 121, 126, 129, 148
Femur: fractures, 47
Fibula: fractures, 83
Finger: fractures, 114
   ligament injuries, 23
   tendon injuries, 119
First Aid facilities, 11
Foot: fractures, 93
   strain, 46
Footballer's ankle, 90
Fractures: see under specific bones
Frequency of injury, 4
Fungal infections, 149

Gait, 99
Gastrocnemius tear, 25
Golfer's elbow, 38
Groin strain, 39

Haemothorax, 140
Hamstrings: pulled, 40
   strains, 142
Hand fractures, 114

INDEX

Head injuries, 15, 121
  prevention, 125
Hernias, 141
Hip: dislocation, 47
Humerus: fractures, 112

Iliotibial band friction, 41
Immediate care, 147
Injury: avoidance, 12
Intracranial haemorrhage, 122

Jumper's knee, 53
Junior leg, 42

Knee: discoid meniscus, 62
  dislocation, 86
  injuries, 83
  ligaments: anterior instability, 74
    anterolateral instability, 77
    anteromedial instability, 75
    combined instability, 80
    injury, 69
    lateral instability, 73
    medial instability, 72
    posterior instability, 73
    posterolateral instability, 78
    rehabilitation, 80
    rotatory instability, 75
    sprain, 69
    stability, 68
  menisci, 55
    functions, 55
    horizontal degeneration, 57
    injury, 55
    lateral tears, 60
    locked knee, 57
    medial tears, 58
    osteoarthrosis knee, 63
    postmeniscectomy problems, 63
    postmeniscectomy rehabilitation, 66
    special problems, 62

Ligament injury, 22
Lumbar spine injuries, 135
Lung: injuries, 139, 141

McLaughlin repair, 25
Magnuson operation, 106
Mallet finger, 119

Mandibular dislocations, 130
Mandibular fractures, 130
March fracture, 97
Medial synovial plica, 52
Medial tibial syndrome, 42
Menisci: see Knee
Metacarpal fractures, 116
Metatarsal fractures, 96, 97
Metatarsal pain, 97
Muscle hernia, 33
Muscle injuries, 32
Myositis ossificans, 33

Nerve damage, 13
Nicholas operation, 76
Nose: injuries, 128

Olecranon: bursae, 119
  fractures, 112
Orbital floor fractures, 130
Osgood–Schlatter's disease, 53
Osteitis pubis, 143
Osteochondritis dissecans, 54

Patella: bipartite, 53
  dislocation, 51
  fracture, 49
Patellar tendon injuries, 25
Pectoral tears, 24, 139
Pellegrini–Stieda's disease, 53
Pelvic injuries, 142
Peroneal tendons: displacement, 28
  sprains, 27
Phalangeal: dislocations, 116
  fractures, 116
Plantar fasciitis, 45
Plantaris rupture, 25
Pneumothorax, 140
Posterior compartment syndromes, 42
Prolapsed intervertebral disc, 138
Pronated foot, 98
Putti–Platt operation, 106

Quadriceps injury, 25

Radius: fractures, 113
Rib: fractures, 139
Rotator cuff tears, 116

INDEX

Sacrum: fractures, 143
Scalp wounds, 122, 148
Scaphoid fractures, 114
Sever's disease, 94
Shin splints, 42
Shoulder: anterior dislocation, 105
  chronic injuries, 36
  dislocation, 103
  injuries, 101
  posterior dislocation, 107
  recurrent, 106
  subluxation, 107
Sinding-Larsen-Johannson disease, 53
Site of injury, 4
Skin: injuries, 146
Skull fractures, 122
Slocum and Larson operation, 78
Soft-tissue injuries: acute, 17
  anti-inflammatory agents, 18
  biochemistry, 18
  chronic, 36
  enzyme preparations, 21
  prophylaxis, 20
  immediate care, 17
  physiotherapy, 21
Spinal injuries, 15, 132
Spondylolisthesis, 137
Spondylolysis, 136
Spring ligament sprain, 46
Stress fractures, 42, 86
Subacromial bursitis, 36
Subconjunctival haemorrhage, 126
Subcutaneous emphysema, 140
Subdural bleeding, 122
Sublingual pain, 97
Sudden death, 7
Superior tibiofibular dislocation, 86
Supracondylar fracture: femur, 49
  humerus, 110
Supraspinatus tears, 117

Tarsus: pain, 94
Tendon injuries: acute, 23
Tendons: snapping, 27
Tennis elbow, 37
Tenosynovitis: ankle, 27
  wrist, 25
Tetanus immunization, 147
Thigh injuries, 47
Thoracic spine injuries, 135
Thumb: fractures, 115
  ligament injuries, 23
Tibial fractures, 83
Tibialis posterior strain, 27
Toe-injury, 96
Toe-nail: care, 149
  ingrowing, 149
Toilet of wounds, 146
Triceps injury, 24

Ulna: fractures, 113
Upper limb injuries, 101

Vascular damage, 13

Warm-up, 12
Wounds, 146

Zygomatic fractures, 130